Exploring Dissociation: Definitions, Development and Cognitive Correlates

Exploring Dissociation: Definitions, Development and Cognitive Correlates has been co-published simultaneously as *Journal of Trauma & Dissociation*, Volume 7, Number 4 2006.

Monographic Separates from the *Journal of Trauma & Dissociation*

For additional information on these and other Haworth Press titles, including descriptions, tables of contents, reviews, and prices, use the QuickSearch catalog at http://www.HaworthPress.com.

Exploring Dissociation: Definitions, Development and Cognitive Correlates, edited by Anne P. DePrince, PhD, and Lisa DeMarni Cromer, PhD (Vol. 7, No. 4, 2006). *A comprehensive overview of the development and conceptualization of dissociation using classic psychological theories of attachment, learning and memory, attention, and intergenerational transmission of trauma, including innovative models and directions for assessment, treatment, and research.*

Acute Reactions to Trauma and Psychotherapy: A Multidisciplinary and International Perspective, edited by Etzel Cardeña, PhD, and Kristin Croyle, PhD (Vol. 6, No. 2, 2005). *"COMPREHENSIVE, INFORMATIVE. . . . CONCISE AND WELL WRITTEN. . . . A wonderful introduction to a summary of current knowledge about acute stress reactions. . . . A USEFUL RESOURCE FOR GRADUATE STUDENTS as well as for trauma and other mental health researchers and practitioners. . . . Covers a wide range of relevant issues, including vulnerabilities and risk factors, diagnosis, effects of acute stress reactions on the brain, treatment, the role of coping, and peritraumatic dissociation. The research reported here crosses a range of potentially traumatic events and experiences such as house fires, terrorist attacks, and burns." (Laurie Anne Pearlman, PhD, Co-Director, Traumatic Stress Institute/Center for Adult & Adolescent Psychotherapy LLC)*

Trauma and Sexuality: The Effects of Childhood Sexual, Physical, and Emotional Abuse on Sexual Identity and Behavior, edited by James A. Chu, MD, and Elizabeth S. Bowman, MD (Vol. 3, No. 4, 2002). *Examines the effects of childhood trauma on sexual orientation and behavior.*

Exploring Dissociation: Definitions, Development and Cognitive Correlates

Anne P. DePrince, PhD
Lisa DeMarni Cromer, PhD
Editors

Exploring Dissociation: Definitions, Development and Cognitive Correlates has been co-published simultaneously as *Journal of Trauma & Dissociation*, Volume 7, Number 4 2006.

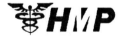

The Haworth Medical Press®
The Haworth Maltreatment & Trauma Press®
Imprints of The Haworth Press, Inc.

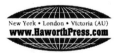

New York • London • Victoria (AU)
www.HaworthPress.com

Published by

The Haworth Medical Press®, 10 Alice Street, Binghamton, NY 13904-1580 USA

The Haworth Medical Press® is an imprint of The Haworth Press, Inc., 10 Alice Street, Binghamton, NY 13904-1580 USA.

Exploring Dissociation: Definitions, Development and Cognitive Correlates has been co-published simultaneously as *Journal of Trauma & Dissociation*, Volume 7, Number 4 2006.

The development, preparation, and publication of this work has been undertaken with great care. However, the publisher, employees, editors, and agents of The Haworth Press and all imprints of The Haworth Press, Inc., including The Haworth Medical Press® and Pharmaceutical Products Press®, are not responsible for any errors contained herein or for consequences that may ensue from use of materials or information contained in this work. With regard to case studies, identities and circumstances of individuals discussed herein have been changed to protect confidentiality. Any resemblance to actual persons, living or dead, is entirely coincidental.

The Haworth Press is committed to the dissemination of ideas and information according to the highest standards of intellectual freedom and the free exchange of ideas. Statements made and opinions expressed in this publication do not necessarily reflect the views of the Publisher, Directors, management, or staff of The Haworth Press, Inc., or an endorsement by them.

Library of Congress Cataloging-in-Publication Data

Exploring dissociation : definitions, development and cognitive correlates / Anne P. DePrince, Lisa DeMarni Cromer, editors.
p. ; cm.
"Co-published simultaneously as Journal of Trauma & Dissociation, volume 7, number 4, 2006."
Includes bibliographical references and index.
ISBN-13: 978-0-7890-3326-0 (hard cover : alk. paper)
ISBN-10: 0-7890-3326-7 (hard cover : alk. paper)
ISBN-13: 978-0-7890-3327-7 (soft cover : alk. paper)
ISBN-10: 0-7890-3327-5 (soft cover : alk. paper)
1. Dissociative disorders–Diagnosis. 2. Condition. I. DePrince, Anne P. II. Cromer, Lisa DeMarni.
[DNLM: 1. Dissociative Disorders–psychology. 2. Cognition. 3. Dissociative Disorders–physiopathology. W1 J0966PK v. 7 no. 4 2006 / WM 173.6 E955 2006]
RC553.D5E97 2006
616.85'23–dc22
2006025370

Indexing, Abstracting & Website/Internet Coverage

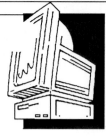

This section provides you with a list of major indexing & abstracting services and other tools for bibliographic access. That is to say, each service began covering this periodical during the year noted in the right column. Most Websites which are listed below have indicated that they will either post, disseminate, compile, archive, cite or alert their own Website users with research-based content from this work. (This list is as current as the copyright date of this publication.)

(continued)

- *Elsevier Eflow-D <http://www.elsevier.com>* 2006
- *Elsevier Scopus <http://www.info.scopus.com>* 2005
- *EMBASE.com (The Power of EMBASE + MEDLINE Combined) (Elsevier) <http://www.embase.com>* 2000
- *EMBASE/Excerpta Medica (Elsevier) <http://www.elsevier.nl>* . . 2000
- *EMCare (Elsevier) <http://www.elsevier.com>* 2006
- *Family & Society Studies Worldwide (NISC USA) <http://www.nisc.com>* 2000
- *Family Violence & Sexual Assault Bulletin* 2006
- *Google <http://www.google.com>* 2004
- *Google Scholar <http://scholar.google.com>* 2004
- *Haworth Document Delivery Center <http://www.HaworthPress.com/journals/dds.asp>* 2000
- *Health & Psychosocial Instruments (HaPI) Database (available through online and as a CD-ROM from Ovid Technologies)* 2001
- *Health Source: Nursing/Academic Edition (EBSCO) <http://www.epnet.com/academic/hsnursing.asp>* 2006
- *Index Copernicus <http://www.indexcopernicus.com>* 2006
- *Index to Periodical Articles Related to Law <http://www.law.utexas.edu>* 2001
- *Internationale Bibliographie der geistes- und sozialwissenschaftlichen Zeitschriftenliteratur . . . See IBZ <http://www.saur.de>* 2001
- *Journal of Social Work Practice "Abstracts Section" <http://www.carfax.co.uk/jsw-ad.htm>* 2000
- *Links@Ovid (via CrossRef targeted DOI links) <http://www.ovid.com>* 2005
- *MANTIS (Manual, Alternative and Natural Therapy) MANTIS is available through three database vendors: Ovid, Dialog & DataStar. In addition it is available for searching through <http://www.healthindex.com>* 2000
- *MEDLINE (National Library of Medicine) <http://www.nlm.nih.gov>* 2005
- *NewJour (Electronic Journals & Newsletters) <http://gort.ucsd.edu/newjour/>* 2006
- *Ovid Linksolver (OpenURL link resolver via CrossRef targeted DOI links) <http://www.linksolver.com>* 2005

(continued)

Special Bibliographic Notes related to special journal issues (separates) and indexing/abstracting:

- indexing/abstracting services in this list will also cover material in any "separate" that is co-published simultaneously with Haworth's special thematic journal issue or DocuSerial. Indexing/abstracting usually covers material at the article/chapter level.
- monographic co-editions are intended for either non-subscribers or libraries which intend to purchase a second copy for their circulating collections.
- monographic co-editions are reported to all jobbers/wholesalers/approval plans. The source journal is listed as the "series" to assist the prevention of duplicate purchasing in the same manner utilized for books-in-series.
- to facilitate user/access services all indexing/abstracting services are encouraged to utilize the co-indexing entry note indicated at the bottom of the first page of each article/chapter/contribution.
- this is intended to assist a library user of any reference tool (whether print, electronic, online, or CD-ROM) to locate the monographic version if the library has purchased this version but not a subscription to the source journal.
- individual articles/chapters in any Haworth publication are also available through the Haworth Document Delivery Service (HDDS).

ALL HAWORTH MEDICAL PRESS BOOKS
AND JOURNALS ARE PRINTED
ON CERTIFIED ACID-FREE PAPER

Exploring Dissociation: Definitions, Development and Cognitive Correlates

CONTENTS

ABOUT THE EDITORS

Anne P. DePrince, PhD, is an Assistant Professor in the Child Clinical and Developmental Cognitive Neuroscience programs in the Department of Psychology at the University of Denver. Her research focuses on the relationship between trauma exposure, emotion, cognitive processes, and posttraumatic distress in both children and adults. DePrince completed her doctoral training at the University of Oregon and her clinical internship at the University of Washington School of Medicine. She is a licensed clinical psychologist in Colorado. DePrince was awarded the 2005 Public Advocacy Award by the International Society for Traumatic Stress Studies. She was co-editor of *Trauma and Cognitive Science: A Meeting of Minds, Science, and Human Experience,* published in 2001.

Lisa DeMarni Cromer, PhD, earned her doctorate in clinical psychology at the University of Oregon. Her research examines the normative development of dissociation from attachment and attention perspectives. Her empirical work also explores factors which impact both reporting of abuse history and biases in others believing reported abuse.

Introduction:
Exploring Dissociation:
Setting the Course

Exploring Dissociation. We have chosen a theme of *exploration* for this volume because successful efforts by dissociation researchers and theorists embody the spirit and skills of explorers. When envisioning an explorer embarking on a trek, one imagines important requisite skills and attitudes. Explorers must be well-grounded in history, drawing on the experience, maps, and map-making tools of those who travelled before. They require curiosity and compassion to motivate their efforts and temper their interpretation of new discoveries and patterning of new knowledge. Indeed, explorers must be open to surprises and to re-evaluating their maps, map-making tools, and travel plans. Thus, exploration is a transactional rather than linear process: new explorations shed new light on previous discoveries and ideas, just as previous ideas affect the development of new plans for future exploration.

As dissociation has garnered greater attention, explorations seeking to describe and understand dissociative phenomena have emerged rapidly in both research and treatment literatures. This surge follows a long history of clinicians and researchers seeking simply to evidence the existence of dissociative phenomena. Early endeavors to document dissociative phenomena were often based on case study descriptions and philosophical musings (see Rieber, 2002 for historical review). Remarkably, many of the ideas of the early theorists who grappled with

[Haworth co-indexing entry note]: "Introduction: Exploring Dissociation: Setting the Course." DePrince, Anne P., and Lisa DeMarni Cromer. Co-published simultaneously in *Journal of Trauma & Dissociation* (The Haworth Medical Press, an imprint of The Haworth Press, Inc.) Vol. 7, No. 4, 2006, pp. 1-6; and: *Exploring Dissociation: Definitions, Development and Cognitive Correlates* (ed: Anne P. DePrince, and Lisa DeMarni Cromer) The Haworth Medical Press, an imprint of The Haworth Press, Inc., 2006, pp. 1-6. Single or multiple copies of this article are available for a fee from The Haworth Document Delivery Service [1-800-HAWORTH, 9:00 a.m. - 5:00 p.m. (EST). E-mail address: docdelivery@haworthpress.com].

Available online at http://jtd.haworthpress.com
doi:10.1300/J229v07n04_01

dissociative phenomena (such as William James, Pierre Janet, G. E. Muller, and Morton Prince) are quite relevant today, including to this volume. For example, Janet talked about divided consciousness, Muller hypothesized inhibition as being related to dissociation, and Morton Prince postulated that more than one explanatory principle would be needed to account for the various facets of dissociation (Rieber, 2002). Thus, current explorations of dissociation can and should be informed by the work of theorists historically.

As the concept of dissociation has gained traction in mainstream psychology and psychiatry in recent years, empirical investigations have enhanced our understanding of the complexity of dissociative phenomena. In the face of these contemporary advancements, the field now faces many theoretical and empirical priorities that are central to continued progress. This volume addresses three of these inter-related priority areas, including efforts to: (1) define dissociation; (2) examine the development of dissociation in terms of both function and etiology; and (3) identify cognitive correlates of dissociation. We will address each of these priority areas in turn.

The first priority area focuses on defining dissociative phenomena. As research and clinical interest in dissociation has increased over the last twenty years, frameworks for organizing dissociative phenomena have developed, at times, in an ad hoc or piecemeal manner. The scope and specificity of the term dissociation has been affected by problems of both over- and under-inclusiveness (see van der Hart, Nihenhuis, Steele, & Brown, 2004). Definitional issues are of central importance to both theory-building and empirical investigations. As the field grows, delineating and clarifying definitional issues, such as whether dissociation is premised to be a state or trait, a continuum or a taxon, an outcome or a mechanism (DePrince & Freyd, in press), is of critical importance for several reasons. Theory building, assessment, and data interpretation all inherently depend on answers to each of those questions: is dissociation a state or trait, a continuum or taxon, an outcome or a mechanism, or some combination? In addition, issues of *construct* validity (i.e., are we measuring the construct, the whole construct and nothing but the construct) affect not only all stages of the research process, but also theory development. Further, only when we have a well-defined construct can we engage in the extraordinarily important work of testing and reconciling competing theories regarding the function, etiology and underlying mechanisms of dissociation. Thus, from early research design efforts up through data interpretation, definitional issues are a core concern.

The second priority area involves developmental issues about the function and etiology of dissociation. Views about the function and etiology of dissociation have expanded in recent years, requiring additional theoretical and empirical attention to distil and extend this literature. As we sort out the various facets and functions of dissociation, definitional issues influence how etiology and function are understood (i.e., whether dissociation is viewed as adaptive or maladaptive, pathological or normative). For example, if dissociation is defined as pathological, views of the function and etiology of dissociative experiences will be linked to that perspective, looking for explanations for a *problem*. In turn, how one views function and etiology acts as a compass for broader theorizing. Further, the framework used to conceptualize etiology acts as a sextant for understanding the role of development and dissociation (and vice versa). For example, to the extent that theorists assume dissociation may play a protective function for children in violent environments, theories about the etiology of symptoms will be tied to those environments. In turn, views of both etiology and function necessarily inform intervention theory and practice.

The third priority area involves identifying cognitive correlates of dissociation. Against the backdrop of developing tools to aid in differential diagnosis and burgeoning exploration into cognitive neuroscience of trauma, investigations into the cognitive correlates of dissociation are a rapidly evolving frontier. Cognitive research and data interpretation are (as all research is) influenced by the paradigm of the researcher. Thus, approaches to examining the cognitive correlates of dissociation tie back to the experimenters' views of the etiology and development of dissociation. For instance, to the extent that dissociative experiences are viewed as pathological in nature, investigations are more likely to focus on deficit-based outcomes. Likewise, to the extent that dissociation is viewed as protective and adaptive, investigations will be geared towards identifying strengths correlated with dissociation. A dialectical view–that dissociation may be both adaptive and harmful (see DePrince & Freyd, in press)–acknowledges both positive and negative correlates of dissociation. As researchers with diverse views about etiology and function of dissociation have ventured into cognitive research, both expected and unexpected findings have emerged. The studies in this volume highlight some interesting, and perhaps surprising, relationships between dissociation (or dissociative styles) and seemingly adaptive aspects of the cognitive flexibility.

Current Volume. Attending to the three priority areas reviewed above, this volume's chapters explore coordinates of definitions, function and etiology, and cognitive correlates of dissociation. Like explorers, the authors build on historical views while synthesizing past theory with contemporary research. Reflecting the spirit of curiosity and intrigue, several chapters in this volume report on unexpected findings regarding dissociation, particularly information processing alterations associated with dissociation. A transactional process is also evident in theoretical chapters that draw on previous theory to innovate and pattern new directions.

Volume Organization. This volume addresses three major issues in dissociation research and theory, respectively: definitions, development (both function and etiology), and cognitive correlates. Volume contributors include international experts on dissociation, cognition, development, and clinical science. This volume offers a compilation of theory and empirical research in a series of chapters that synthesize existing literature with advanced study. The contributors also pose innovative questions about correlates of dissociation. Across articles the contributors offer rich discussions of previous research to inform new viewpoints. This volume is poised to galvanize discussion about models of dissociation, particularly innovative views of dissociation, cognition and development.

Mapping Definitions. The first two chapters focus on defining dissociative phenomena. Brown's opens the volume by building on recent work in defining a bipartite model of dissociation. Expanding on Holmes' and colleagues (2005) model, Brown delineates two qualitatively distinct forms of dissociation: detachment and compartmentalization. These different phenomena are argued to have different mechanisms, base rates, and treatment implications. Dorahy's chapter extends an important discussion of definitional issues in the literature. Dorahy proposes that a dissociative processing style precedes dissociative experiences, and draws critical distinctions between cognitive styles, dissociative phenomena, and correlates of dissociative phenomena. Dorahy's article also raises important issues about the function of dissociation, particularly in the face of perceived threat.

Mapping Development. Extending themes about both function and etiology, chapters by Liotti, and by Chu and DePrince, address questions of developmental etiology. Liotti navigates through the attachment literature providing important etiological and intervention considerations. Chu and DePrince embark upon empirically investigating parenting (including parent dissociation and trauma exposure) and parenting behaviors that influence the intergenerational transmission of mothers' dissociation to children.

Mapping Cognitive Correlates. Finally, surprising consequences of dissociation are explored across three manuscripts: Holmes and colleagues, de Ruiter and colleagues, and Cromer and colleagues. Holmes and colleagues take the reader back to dissociation's early roots in hypnosis to experimentally test the impact of state dissociation on intrusive memories for a traumatic film. de Ruiter and collaborators utilize brain imaging experimental data to explore learning styles and cognitive elaboration in nonpathological dissociation. Venturing into relatively new territory, these studies add to only a handful of others (e.g., DePrince & Freyd, 1999; Elzinga, deBeurs, Sergeant, vanDyck, & Phaf, 2000) that document relative cognitive strengths associated with dissociation, versus *dis*abilities. Finally, Cromer and colleagues extend the scope of their investigation of dissociation to children as young as 5 years old, finding that Muller's suggestion made over a century ago, that dissociation is related to inhibition, may indeed have roots in childhood.

Summary. This volume brings together researchers of many theoretical and empirical perspectives to comment on three central issues in the field through both theoretical and empirical papers. Together, these papers transact to inform, challenge, and synthesize ideas from each priority area (definition, development, and cognitive correlates). The chapters are by no means an exhaustive review of the exciting breadth and depth reflected in the dissociation literature; however, we hope these contributions will galvanize interest and discussion in pushing explorations of dissociation forward.

Anne P. DePrince, PhD
Department of Psychology
University of Denver
Denver, CO 80208

Lisa DeMarni Cromer, PhD
Department of Psychology
University of Oregon
Eugene, OR 97403

REFERENCES

DePrince, A.P. & Freyd, J.J. (2006). Trauma-induced dissociation. *PTSD: Science & Practice–A Comprehensive Handbook.* M.J. Friedman, T.M. Keane & P.A. Resick (Eds.). Guilford Press, Manuscript in press.
DePrince, A.P. and Freyd, J.J. (1999). Dissociation, attention, and memory. *Psychological Science, 10*, 449-452.

Elzinga, B.M., de Beurs, E., Sergeant, J.A., Van Dyck, R., & Phaf, R.H. (2000). Dissociative style and directed forgetting. *Cognitive Therapy and Research, 24,* 279-295.

Rieber, R. W. (2002). Multiplicity of the Mind and the Duality of the Brain: Can You Have It Both Ways, *History of Psychiatry,* March. Retrieved May 9, 2006 from: http://web.jjay.cuny.edu/~jpr/can%20you%20have%20it%20both%20ways.doc

van der Hart, O., Nijenhuis, E., Steele, K., & Brown, D. (2004). Trauma-related dissociation: Conceptual clarity lost and found. *Australian and New Zealand Journal of Psychiatry, 38,* 906-914.

doi:10.1300/J229v07n04_01

Different Types of "Dissociation" Have Different Psychological Mechanisms

Richard J. Brown, PhD, ClinPsyD

SUMMARY. The term "dissociation" has been used to describe a wide range of psychological and psychiatric phenomena. The popular conception of dissociation describes it as a unitary phenomenon, with only quantitative differences in severity between the various dissociative conditions. More recently, it has been argued that the available evidence is more consistent with a model that identifies at least two distinct categories of dissociative phenomena–"detachment" and "compartmentalization"–that have different definitions, mechanisms and treatment implications (Holmes, Brown, Mansell, Fearon, Hunter, Frasquilho & Oakley 2005). This paper presents evidence for this bipartite model of dissociation, followed by definitions and descriptions of detachment and compartmentalization. Possible psychological mechanisms underlying these phenomena are then discussed, with particular emphasis on the nature of compartmentalization in conversion disorder, hypnosis, dissociative amnesia and dissociative identity disorder. doi:10.1300/J229v07n04_02 *[Article copies available for a fee from The Haworth Document Delivery Service: 1-800-HAWORTH. E-mail address: <docdelivery@haworthpress.com> Website: <http://www.HaworthPress.com> © 2006 by The Haworth Press, Inc. All rights reserved.]*

Richard J. Brown is affiliated with the Academic Division of Clinical Psychology, University of Manchester.

Address correspondence to: Dr. Richard J. Brown, Academic Division of Clinical Psychology, University of Manchester, Rawnsley Building, Manchester Royal Infirmary, Oxford Road, Manchester, M13 9WL, UK (E-mail: richard.james.brown@manchester.ac.uk).

[Haworth co-indexing entry note]: "Different Types of "Dissociation" Have Different Psychological Mechanisms." Brown, Richard J. Co-published simultaneously in *Journal of Trauma & Dissociation* (The Haworth Medical Press, an imprint of The Haworth Press, Inc.) Vol. 7, No. 4, 2006, pp. 7-28; and: *Exploring Dissociation: Definitions, Development and Cognitive Correlates* (ed: Anne P. DePrince, and Lisa DeMarni Cromer) The Haworth Medical Press, an imprint of The Haworth Press, Inc., 2006, pp. 7-28. Single or multiple copies of this article are available for a fee from The Haworth Document Delivery Service [1-800-HAWORTH, 9:00 a.m. - 5:00 p.m. (EST). E-mail address: docdelivery@haworthpress.com].

Available online at http://jtd.haworthpress.com
© 2006 by The Haworth Press, Inc. All rights reserved.
doi:10.1300/J229v07n04_02

KEYWORDS. Dissociation, detachment, compartmentalization, bipartite model

INTRODUCTION

When the term "dissociation"[1] was originally popularised in the 19th century, it was used to refer to a putative mental mechanism underlying a relatively circumscribed set of clinical phenomena (Van der Hart & Dorahy, in press). Since the renaissance of the concept in the 1970s, however, and the growth of contemporary theories (e.g., Hilgard, 1977) concerning the nature of this mental mechanism, the number of phenomena thought to be attributable to dissociation has expanded considerably. As a result, the dissociation label is now applied to an extraordinary range of psychological symptoms, states and processes (see Figure 1; Cardeña, 1994).

On the face of it, this expansion of the dissociative domain (Cardeña, 1994) appears to be justified by the widespread view that these different phenomena described above are produced by a common psychological mechanism (i.e., dissociation), characterised by a breakdown in mental integration (e.g., Bernstein & Putnam, 1986; Dell, 2006). According to this "unitary" model, these phenomena are all qualitatively similar, with the differences between them being accounted for by the "amount" of

FIGURE 1. Psychological symptoms, states and processes associated with the dissociation label

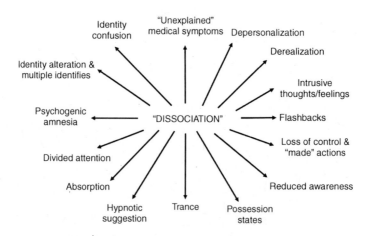

dissociation involved in each case. This idea is embodied in the concept of the so-called dissociative continuum (Figure 2) and forms the basis for the Dissociative Experiences Scale (DES; Bernstein & Putnam, 1986), which is commonly used to estimate individual differences in "trait" dissociation. The model is also apparent in the DSM-IV definition of dissociation, which identifies it as ". . . a disruption in the usually integrated functions of consciousness, memory, identity or perception of the environment" (p. 477; APA, 1994). The unitary model is able to account for a large body of research findings demonstrating that the DES scores of different clinical groups vary as predicted, with the most disabling conditions (such as DID) being associated with the highest DES scores (see Van Ijzendoorn & Schuengel, 1996). In addition, the model provides a parsimonious and accessible account of the available clinical data and is therefore intuitively appealing to both clinicians and patients.

Despite the appeal of the unitary model, it is not without its critics (see, e.g., Cardeña, 1994; Frankel, 1990, 1994; Van der Hart, Nijenhuis, Steele & Brown, 2004). According to Frankel (1990, 1994), for example, the dissociation concept has been over-extended to encompass almost any kind of symptom involving an alteration in consciousness or a loss of mental or behavioural control. Similarly, Holmes et al. (2005) have argued that the unitary model is based on a definition of dissociation that is too broad and which obscures fundamental differences between the various phenomena that it encompasses. If valid, this argument has far-reaching implications. Empirically, it implies that re-

FIGURE 2. Hypothetical dissociative continuum (not to scale). N. B. The inclusion of both states and disorders on a single dimensional scale is deliberate in order to illustrate the assumption underlying the unitary model, *viz.* that different dissociative states and conditions can be regarded as involving different "amounts" of dissociation

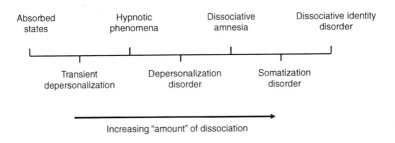

searchers need to move beyond simply recruiting generic groups of patients with "dissociative disorders" and instead focus on the specific symptoms or symptom clusters in question. Clinically, it indicates that different types of treatment may be required for different dissociative problems, and that the "one-size-fits-all" approach implied by the unitary model is invalid.

Numerous previous theorists have attempted to address the confusion caused by the unitary model by identifying different and separate "types" of dissociation (Cardeña, 1994; Allen, 2001; Putnam, 1997; Brown, 2002a; Van der Kolk & Fisler, 1995). Holmes et al. (2005) provide a summary position based on these previous theories, arguing that the available evidence is consistent with a model that distinguishes between two qualitatively different kinds of phenomena–"detachment" and "compartmentalization" (following Allen, 2001)–each with distinct definitions, mechanisms and treatment implications. In the first half of this paper, I will describe the Holmes et al. (2005) model, providing definitions and descriptions of detachment and compartmentalization, as well as evidence supporting a distinction between these phenomena. In the second half, I will elaborate on the Holmes et al. (2005) model by relating it to a recent account of the cognitive mechanisms underlying compartmentalization (Brown, 2002a, 2004; Brown & Oakley, 2004).

EVIDENCE FOR TWO TYPES OF PATHOLOGICAL "DISSOCIATION"

Although research investigating total scores on the DES seems to support a unitary model of dissociation, factor analytic studies of the measure are more consistent with a multifactorial account. Numerous studies have found that the DES has a complex factor structure with at least three underlying factors (e.g., Carlson, Putnam, Ross et al., 1991; Ross, Ellason & Anderson, 1995; Frischolz, Braun, Sachs, et al., 1991; Ross, Joshi & Currie, 1991). Almost invariably, such studies have identified separate factors for absorption, depersonalization-derealization, and amnesia related items, suggesting that these three forms of "dissociation" do not belong to the same category of phenomena. One possible explanation for this pattern of findings is that absorption, depersonalization-derealization, and amnesia occur at different rates in the population, producing a misleading multi-factorial solution when the DES is factor-analyzed (Bernstein, Ellason, Ross & Vanderlinden, 2001). This would be consistent with the widespread view that absorption is a common and non-pathological phenomenon experienced by most people to varying degrees, unlike "pathological" forms of dissociation such as amnesia, depersonalization-derealization and identity alteration (e.g., Waller, Putnam & Carlson, 1996). While this could explain why a separate absorption factor was identified in the Bernstein et al. (2001) study, it is less clear how it could account for the identification of separate amnesia and depersonalization-derealization factors, particularly as there was no evidence that these two had different base-rates in the general population sample that was assessed.

According to Holmes et al. (2005), the statistical separation of amnesia and depersonalization-derealization items on the DES reflects the fact that these phenomena belong to two qualitatively different categories of experience—compartmentalization and detachment respectively—that can be distinguished both empirically and conceptually. Consistent with this, Holmes et al. (2005) point to a number of other studies suggesting that depersonalization and derealization can be separated from amnesia and other "dissociative" phenomena, such as somatoform symptoms[2] and comparable experiences produced using hypnotic suggestion. Research on depersonalization disorder, for example, demonstrates that medically unexplained (i.e., somatoform) symptoms are relatively rare in this group (Baker et al., 2003). Similarly, patients with depersonalization disorder fall in the average range on a sub-scale of the DES made up of amnesia-related items, despite having elevated scores on a depersonalization-derealization sub-scale (Simeon et al., 2003). Furthermore, depersonalization and derealization are relatively uncommon in patients with medically unexplained symptoms (Brown, Schrag & Trimble, 2005). In contrast, patients with amnesia and dissociative disorders such as DID often report somatoform symptoms (Saxe et al., 1994; Nijenhuis, 2004). Patients with somatoform symptoms often yield low scores on the DES, however, because the scale has relatively few items pertaining to amnesia and other examples of compartmentalization (Brown, 2005). Indeed, the somatoform dissociation questionnaire (SDQ-20) was developed to rectify this omission in the DES (Nijenhuis, 2004).

Probably the strongest support for the distinction between depersonalization-derealization and other types of "dissociative" phenomena comes from research addressing their mechanisms. This will be considered in some detail below, following definitions and descriptions of detachment and compartmentalization as described in the Holmes et al. (2005) model.

DETACHMENT

Definition and Description of Detachment

Holmes et al. (2005) define detachment as *an altered state of consciousness characterized by a sense of separation (or 'detachment') from aspects of everyday experience* (see also Cardeña, 1994; Allen, 2001). The sense of detachment may relate to the individual's emotional experience (as in emotional numbing), their sense of self (as in some depersonalization phenomena), their body (as in out-of-body phenomena), or the world around them (as in derealization; see Table 1). The phenomena may occur in isolation although they commonly co-occur. In each case, the individual's sense of reality testing during the detachment experience is preserved. Phenomenological descriptions of detachment include an absence or alteration of emotional experience, feelings of being "spaced out," "disconnected," "unreal" or "in a dream," a sense of being an outside observer of one's body, and perceptions of the external world as flat, lifeless and "strange" (Noyes & Kletti, 1977; Steinberg, 1994; Butler, Duran, Jasiukaitis, Koopman & Spiegel, 1996; Allen, Console & Lewis, 1999; Sierra & Berrios, 2001; Baker et al., 2003). In some cases, detached states are associated with memory disturbances and amnesia (Allen et al., 1999). On the face of it, detachment-related memory dysfunction can be difficult to distinguish from amnesia as a compartmentalization phenomenon. According to the Holmes et al. (2005) model, however, the mechanisms responsible for detachment-related memory loss are different to those operating in compartmentalization (see below).

Detachment phenomena may manifest as a disorder in their own right, as in depersonalization disorder, or in the context of another con-

TABLE 1. Detachment and compartmentalization phenomena

Detachment phenomena	Compartmentalization phenomena
Emotional numbing	Unexplained neurological symptoms
Depersonalization	Hypnotic phenomena
Derealization	"Made" actions
Out-of-body experiences	Multiple identities
Amnesia due to encoding deficit	Amnesia due to retrieval deficit
Identity confusion*	

* Identity confusion is a non-specific symptom that can be associated with either detachment or compartmentalization

dition, such as an anxiety or affective disorder (Hunter, Sierra & David, 2004). Detachment is also commonly experienced during, or immediately after, traumatic events, a phenomenon known as "peri-traumatic dissociation," which is a defining feature of acute stress disorder (ASD) in DSM-IV.[3] In addition, many individuals report mild and transient detachment experiences during periods of fatigue, intoxication or stress. As such, detachment phenomena can be arranged on a continuum of increasing distress and disability, ranging from mild and non-pathological experiences of detachment to extremely disabling symptoms, such as those seen in depersonalization disorder.

In the original Holmes et al. (2005) model, all depersonalization phenomena were regarded as examples of detachment. In the formulation of the model that is outlined here, however, "made" actions, which are routinely identified as examples of depersonalization, are regarded as cases of compartmentalization (see below).

Mechanisms of Detachment

Holmes et al. (2005) follow Sierra and Berrios (1998) in assuming that detached states result from a hard-wired biological defence mechanism evolved to minimize the potentially debilitating effects of extreme affect in threatening situations. By this view, detachment arises when an increase in anxiety causes the medial prefrontal cortex to inhibit emotional processing by the limbic system, thereby reducing sympathetic output (Sierra & Berrios, 1998). The result is a state devoid of emotional experience that facilitates adaptive behavior in the face of threat. Although this detached state is adaptive in the short term, it may be highly aversive and debilitating if it persists over time, as in depersonalization disorder. Hunter, Phillips, Chalder, Sierra and David (2003) suggest that chronicity may develop when the individual misinterprets the state of detachment itself as a threat (e.g., of impending mental breakdown), perpetuating anxiety and emotional inhibition.

There is a growing body of evidence in favour of this account of the mechanisms of detachment. It is well documented, for example, that depersonalization and derealization are commonly associated with anxiety, both normal (e.g., Sterlini & Bryant, 2002) and pathological (e.g., Cassano et al., 1989; Simeon, Gross, Guralnik, Stein, Schmeidler & Hollander, 1997; Marshall, Schneier, Lin, Simpson, Vermes & Leibowitz, 2000). Compared to normal and anxious control participants, depersonalization disorder patients also show significantly reduced skin conductance amplitudes and increased skin conductance latencies (both measures of emotional reactivity) to unpleasant stimuli, but not to neutral, unpleasant or non-specific stimuli (Sierra et al., 2002). Similarly, compared to anxious and normal controls, depersonalization disorder patients show reduced neural responses in brain regions typically activated by emotional stimuli (insula and occipto-temporal cortex) and increased neural responses in regions associated with emotional regulation (right ventral prefrontal cortex) when exposed to aversive pictures (Phillips et al., 2001). Other evidence provides indirect support for the idea that detachment is associated with a hard-wired neurophysiological profile, including the stability of depersonalization disorder semiology over time (Sierra & Berrios, 2001) and the occurrence of detachment phenomena in neurological conditions and drug states (Lambert, Sierra, Phillips & David, 2002).

COMPARTMENTALIZATION

Definition and Description of Compartmentalization

Following Cardeña (1994), Holmes et al. (2005) provide the following definition of compartmentalization phenomena: (i) the phenomenon involves a deficit in the ability to deliberately control processes or actions that would normally be amenable to such control; (ii) the deficit cannot be overcome by an act of will; (iii) the deficit is reversible, at least in principle; and (iv) it can be shown that the apparently disrupted functions are operating normally and continue to influence cognition, emotion and action. This definition encompasses dissociative amnesia, fugue, DID and the various physical symptoms characteristic of the conversion disorders and some somatoform disorders (e.g., somatization disorder; for other examples of "somatoform dissociation" see Nijenhuis, 2004). Similar phenomena (i.e., amnesia, anaesthesia, pseudohallucinations, motor disturbances, etc.) that can be produced using hypnotic suggestion are also included in this category (see Oakley, 1999; Brown, 2004). In addition, unlike the original formulation of the Holmes et al. (2005) model, the current account of compartmentalization also encompasses actions that the individual does not feel they are controlling (so-called "made" actions; Dell, 2004), which are typically regarded as examples of depersonalization (see, e.g., Steinberg, 1994).

Compartmentalization phenomena can also be regarded as occupying their own continuum of distress and disability, ranging from nonpathological experiences produced using hypnotic suggestion, through milder pathological states such as transient amnesias and conversion disorders, to chronic and extremely disabling conditions like somatization disorder and DID. In each case, the apparently disrupted functions are said to be "compartmentalized."

Rather than providing a detailed account of the psychological mechanisms underlying compartmentalization, Holmes et al. (2005) describe laboratory examples that illustrate this phenomenon and distinguish it from detachment. Probably the most compelling empirical demonstration of pathological compartmentalization is an innovative study by Kuyk, Spinhoven and Van Dyck (1999). Kuyk et al. (1999) compared a group of patients with amnesia following generalized non-epileptic seizures (NES; a form of compartmentalization according to the current scheme) and a group with amnesia following generalized epileptic seizures (ES). Participants in both groups were hypnotized some time after a seizure and given suggestions for the recovery of memories concerning events occurring during the ictus. All information recovered using this procedure was corroborated independently. On this basis, Kuyk et al. (1999) found that 85% of their NES patients recalled information about the seizure for which they were previously amnesic, compared to 0% of patients in the ES group. The findings of this study clearly demonstrate that the NES patients had encoded information about events occurring during their seizure, but the compartmentalization of this information within the cognitive system had rendered it unavailable for deliberate retrieval. Hypnotic suggestion had later been able to overturn this retrieval failure, allowing recall to take place. The ES patients, in contrast, did not recover ictal information following hypnosis presumably because a generalized brain dysfunction had prevented material from being encoded during the seizure (Brown, 2002b). Following Allen et al. (1999), we assume that amnesia associated with a period of profound detachment also reflects an encoding failure, thereby distinguishing it from the inability to retrieve stored information in amnesia associated with compartmentalization. At present, this remains a conceptual assumption that requires empirical validation.

Other published demonstrations of compartmentalization can be found in single case studies of so-called implicit perception (Kihlstrom, 1992) in conversion disorder patients. Bryant and McConkey (1989), for example, tested a patient (DB) with unilateral conversion blindness using a forced-choice visual decision paradigm. In this, DB was presented with three visual stimuli (triangles) to his affected eye and he was asked to generate a response indicating which of the three stimuli was oriented differently to the other two. Using this procedure, Bryant and

McConkey (1989) showed that DB responded correctly on 74% of the trials, an above-chance response rate indicating that his performance was influenced by the visual information available, despite the fact that he continued to report a lack of visual experience in his affected eye. This is clearly consistent with the definition of compartmentalization outlined above. DB's response rate also improved following feedback suggesting that his performance was affected by the visual information and improved further still when he was given instructions designed to increase his motivation. These latter findings indicate that the nature of the compartmentalization associated with DB's blindness was relatively fluid and subject to modification through top-down influences. Other single-case studies of implicit perception associated with compartmentalization are described in Kihlstrom (1992).

Although the study reported by Kuyk et al. (1999) and single case studies such as that of Bryant and McConkey (1989) provide compelling examples of compartmentalization, they do not provide a detailed explanation of the mechanisms underlying these phenomena, which is largely lacking from the Holmes et al. (2005) model. In a bid to address this issue, the second half of this paper extends the Holmes et al. (2005) model by relating it to the integrative cognitive model described by Brown (2002a, 2004; Brown & Oakley, 2004; also Oakley, 1999a, b), which has been used recently to account for a range of compartmentalization phenomena.

Mechanisms of Compartmentalization

The integrative cognitive model was originally developed as an account of the mechanisms underlying certain somatoform symptoms as well as comparable experiences produced using hypnotic suggestion, both of which are examples of compartmentalization according to Holmes et al. (2005). The integrative model is based on the assumption that these phenomena result from subtle disturbances in the processes underlying consciousness and mental control. To this end, the model provides a detailed account of the cognitive structures and processes associated with normal consciousness and control, which is then applied to atypical cases such as compartmentalization phenomena.

Consciousness and Cognitive Control

The basic cognitive architecture according to this approach is presented in Figure 3. In line with much cognitive theorising, the model

FIGURE 3. Structures and processes involved in the generation of consciousness and control of cognition and action

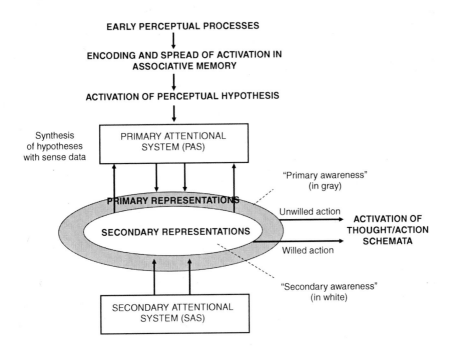

assumes that the contents of consciousness represent a working interpretation of the environment that is generated for the control of cognition and action. In this architecture, the contents of consciousness are generated at a relatively late stage in the processing chain, following extensive pre-attentive analysis of incoming information (Velmans, 2000). In the first instance, the receipt of sensory information triggers simple perceptual analyses that represent its basic features (Kosslyn, 1996). The resulting representations are then encoded in memory, triggering a parallel spread of activation through related representations within memory (Logan, 1988). This spread of activation in associative memory acts as an interpretive process (Sloman, 1996) that produces a number of possible "hypotheses" about the input based on previous experience (Marcel, 1983). These hypotheses are repeatedly sampled by a primary attentional system (PAS), which selects one of the hypotheses as the most appropriate account of the current situation. The PAS then integrates the chosen hypothesis with relevant sensory information, producing multi-modal units or *primary representations*. These primary representations correspond to the basic contents of consciousness and provide a working model of the world that can be used to guide action. Primary representations serve as input to a hierarchical network of behavioral programs or "schemata" (cf. Hilgard, 1977; Norman & Shallice, 1986) that describe the processing operations required for the execution of specific acts. At the top of this hierarchy are high-level programs corresponding to general situations such as "driving a car" or "going to a restaurant." Within each of these high-level programs are simpler schemata corresponding to different acts within that situation, such as "reversing" or "ordering food." Each of these schemata has even simpler sub-programs describing the various elements of the act (e.g., "changing gear" or "reading the menu") and so on. These programs are activated to varying degrees by the current primary representation. When a threshold level of activation is reached, the program is triggered automatically and the associated behavior is executed using the primary representation as a template of the current environment. This behavior will then run until completion unless it is impeded or inhibited by other information in the system. This automatic activation of schemata provides the system with an efficient way of controlling processing in routine situations and is comparable to the contention scheduling mechanism described by Norman and Shallice (1986). Processes controlled by the automatic activation of schemata are regarded as voluntary but *unwilled* (cf. Jahanshahi & Frith, 1998). Processing at this level is perceived as effortless and is associated with an intuitive or pre-reflective subjective character labelled *primary awareness.*

In cases where the network of behavioral programs is unable to produce adaptive behaviour, such as novel situations, a secondary attentional system (SAS)[4] may intervene to bias the activation levels of relevant programs. The SAS operates via general-purpose problem-solving algorithms, the construction of goals (or *secondary representations*) and the analysis and manipulation of primary representations. Primary representations that are subjected to focal-attentive processing (Velmans, 2000) by the SAS are in the foreground of perceptual experience; those that are not currently being processed by the SAS form the perceptual background. Processing controlled by the SAS is *willed* (cf. Jahanshahi & Frith, 1998), effortful, deliberate and associated with a subjective character of self-awareness (i.e., an awareness of being awareness) labelled *secondary awareness.*

This model of the cognitive architecture has important implications for the explanation of somatoform symptoms, hypnotic experiences and other types of compartmentalization phenomena. In particular, the model assumes that sensation and the contents of experience need not match, as the latter are shaped by both sensory and memorial information and may therefore be "over-determined" by memory. Any discrepancies between sensation and experience will not be experienced directly by the individual (although they may be inferred *post hoc*) as the processes involved in the creation of experience are unavailable to introspection. As a result, the individual may engage in behaviour that is consistent with the interpretation of events that is currently dominating their experience, irrespective of whether that interpretation is correct. The model also assumes that many, if not most, behaviours are governed by the automatic activation of behavioral programs (i.e., the PAS) rather than via deliberate selection and control by the individual (i.e., the SAS). As such, many complex behaviours can be performed with minimal representation in conscious experience (or, at least, self-conscious experience; cf. Hilgard, 1977). In addition, there can be significant discrepancies between automatically controlled behaviours and goals in self-awareness.

Compartmentalization Phenomena and Incongruous Memory Retrieval

According to the current approach, all compartmentalization phenomena are similar in that they arise from disturbances in the memory retrieval processes associated with the construction of consciousness and/or automatic control of action. By this view, the nature of specific compartmentalization phenomena will vary according to the type of information (or "rogue representation") involved in the retrieval process. Phenomena characterised by a distortion in conscious experience, such as unexplained (or suggested) pain, pseudohallucinations, sensory alterations/loss, etc., arise from the retrieval of inappropriate (i.e., inconsistent with sense data) perceptual hypotheses from memory during the creation of primary representations by the PAS. The result is a compelling distortion in the perceptual world related to the content of the inappropriately selected memory. Phenomena characterised by a loss of deliberate control over processes that are normally amenable to such control, such as unexplained (or suggested) paralysis, seizures, urinary retention, amnesia, etc., result from the automatic selection of inappropriate behavioral programs corresponding to the experience in question.

Thus, amnesia may result from a program specifying the inhibition of certain memory content, while a paralysis may arise from a program inhibiting bodily movements. Behavioral programs may be activated either directly or through the creation of a distorted primary representation that is consistent with the program content (e.g., an experience of stiffness in the arm triggering a program inhibiting arm movement).

Broadly speaking, then, compartmentalization phenomena arise when the cognitive system misinterprets information in memory (i.e., rogue representations) as the most appropriate account of, or response to, current circumstances. Rogue representations can be acquired from a number of different sources, both internal (e.g., direct experience of the symptom, imagery/fantasy, verbal auto-suggestion) and external (e.g., exposure to symptoms in others, media images, hetero-suggestion; see Brown, 2004; also Johnson & Raye, 1981). In each case, the symptom is generated at a late stage in the processing chain, either during the construction of primary representations by the PAS or via the automatic activation of behavioral programs by those representations. As these processes operate prior to focal processing by self-conscious systems (i.e., the SAS), the individual experiences a subjectively compelling deficit that is outside their willed control. Importantly, the apparently damaged functions or systems operate normally prior to attentional selection by the PAS: it is only the conscious representation of these systems' output that is disrupted. Moreover, the affected systems can still influence on-going thought and action by their effect on other, non-affected, aspects of processing. In these senses, symptoms generated in this way can be regarded as archetypal examples of compartmentalization.

The misinterpretation underlying compartmentalization is driven by the over-activation of rogue representations in memory; as such, any factor that increases this activation will increase the likelihood of a rogue representation being selected and therefore moderate the occurrence of compartmentalization (see Brown, 2004; Brown & Oakley, 2004). In some cases, this may be cognitive factors such as symptom checking, catastrophic thinking and illness worry/rumination; in others, motivational factors (e.g., avoidance of alternative memory content) may be central.

At present, the integrative cognitive model has been applied to medically unexplained symptoms (including amnesia and pseudohallucinations) but not other forms of pathological compartmentalization such as "made" actions. On the face of it, the sense of involuntariness that accompanies such actions is akin to that associated with apparently automatic behaviours in the hypnotic context (the so-called "classic suggestion effect"). According to Brown and Oakley (2004), this phenomenon arises when an unwilled act (i.e., one governed by the automatic activation of a behavioral program) is misinterpreted as coming from an external source, due to certain information about that act within the cognitive system. In some cases, this information may be the absence of an advance prediction about the sensory consequences of the act (see Blakemore, Wolpert & Frith, 2002; Blakemore, Oakley & Frith, 2003) and/or the activation of a goal specifying that the behavior should be experienced as involuntary (Kirsch & Lynn, 1997). In others, it may be the activation of a goal that is inconsistent with the act, particularly if the individual is motivated not to experience it as their own due to its "unacceptability."

The Working Self and Compartmentalization in Dissociative Amnesia and DID

One of the basic assumptions of the Holmes et al. (2005) model is that similar mechanism are operating in all compartmentalization phenomena. How might the integrative cognitive model account for the various symptoms of DID, such as the occurrence of multiple identities and inter-identity amnesia? Although an extensive discussion of this issue is beyond the scope of this article, some theoretical speculations are in order. As with other aspects of the model, the most appropriate approach is to begin by understanding the nature and development of the self under normal circumstances. The self-memory system model of Conway and Pleydell-Pearce (2000; also Conway, 2005) provides a number of important insights into this process that could be used to develop the integrative cognitive model in this respect. According to Conway and Pleydell-Pearce (2000), the self (or *working self* in their terminology) consists of a set of hierarchically-organized goals in working memory constructed to reduce discrepancies between current and desired states of the system; these discrepancies are associated with negative emotional experiences, which provide the motivating force behind goal development and maintenance. The working self has access to an autobiographical knowledge base that represents information about previous events that pertain to system goals. The retrieval of individual autobiographical memories occurs when a stable pattern of activation develops within the autobiographical knowledge base that is linked to current goals in the working self. This may occur through the creation of a deliberate retrieval plan by the working self or via direct activation of the knowledge base by cues from the environment.

Although developed for quite different purposes, the model of Conway and Pleydell-Pearce's (2000) is consistent with many aspects of the integrative cognitive model described above. Thus, the goal hierarchy that constitutes Conway and Pleydell-Pearce's working self would be an important aspect of the control structures that make up the secondary attentional system, whereas the autobiographical knowledge base would be one part of associative memory. By this view, autobiographical memories will be retrieved when their activation patterns in associative memory are sufficient for them to be selected by the PAS during the creation of primary representations. This may occur via the creation of new retrieval programs by the SAS, the activation of old retrieval programs by primary representations, or the direct activation of associative memory by environmental cues.

One important feature of the Conway and Pleydell-Pearce model that is not explicit in the integrative cognitive model is the idea that autobiographical memory retrieval is strongly constrained by the goals of the working self. According to Conway and Pleydell-Pearce (2000), one important goal of the working self is to limit the retrieval of autobiographical memories that may be destabilizing to the system, such as those that are associated with strong affect and/or highlight discrepancies between goals and knowledge. The working self does this by creating retrieval programs that specify inhibition of memory content of this sort, which remains compartmentalized in the system. Conway and Pleydell-Pearce suggest that this may be one route to the development of traumatic amnesia in PTSD, an idea that could conceivably be extended to all forms of dissociative memory loss. The account of dissociative amnesia provided by the integrative cognitive model is entirely consistent with this notion if one assumes that the process is similar whether the inhibitory retrieval program (i.e., rogue representation) is established in memory or created on-line by the SAS.[5]

The idea that self goals determine what is available for autobiographical recall could also help account for the occurrence of dissociative amnesia in patients with DID, although a more complex explanation is probably required here. In normal circumstances, the working self will have a high degree of internal consistency, such that the various goals within the structure are mutually compatible. In cases where there is a discrepancy between conflicting goals (e.g., the goal to develop a romantic relationship vs. the goal to avoid rejection at all costs), negative affect (e.g., anxiety) will arise. This affect can be managed by reducing the discrepancy between the conflicting goals, either through adaptive (e.g., adopting a more realistic goal in relation to rejection) or maladaptive means (e.g., avoiding romantic relationships). In chaotic or traumatic environments, however, it may be impossible to reduce discrepancies between basic behavioral goals (e.g., the goal to be close to attachment figures and the goal to avoid physical or emotional pain). One way for the cognitive system to manage the resulting anxiety would be to prevent the simultaneous activation of the conflicting goals. If this were to happen often enough, separate goal hierarchies (or working selves) could develop over time, each comprising the goals and subgoals that were co-active with the conflicting goal in question. Each goal hierarchy would have access to the autobiographical memories associated with its component goals, while memories associated with the conflicting goal would either be inhibited or unavailable due to the lack of relevant links in the knowledge base.[6] Such a fragmented goal hierarchy could account for the gaps in time experienced by many patients with DID, as well as the occurrence of multiple identities with interidentity amnesia. The characteristic behavioral pattern of each identity would reflect the type of goals that make up the goal-hierarchy in question. It is likely that these will be organised around fundamental behavioral goals or action tendencies such as those described by Nijenhuis, Van der Hart and Steele (2004).

According to this account, the compartmentalization operating in less pathological phenomena such as simple conversion disorders or circumscribed dissociative amnesias involves a separation (or "dissociation") between different levels of processing within the cognitive system (i.e., the results of low level processing are separated from the SAS by the PAS). In DID, the compartmentalization is not only between the PAS and SAS, but also within SAS structures themselves. In many ways, this distinction is similar to that between the different levels of structural dissociation (i.e., primary and secondary vs. tertiary) in the Nijenhuis et al. (2004) model.

This account of compartmentalization in DID is clearly both speculative and in need of further development. Nevertheless, it provides some indication of how the symptoms of DID might be understood using cognitive models such as those of Conway and Pleydell-Pearce (2000) and Brown (2004), suggesting that this may be a fruitful avenue for future investigation.

IMPLICATIONS AND CONCLUSIONS

The model of Holmes et al. (2005) has a number of important empirical and clinical implications. In particular, the model emphasises that total scores on the DES may not be the most useful way of describing the "dissociative" tendencies of subject groups and that sub-scales of the DES, or more specific measures of detachment and/or compartmentalization, may be more appropriate for research or clinical purposes. Similarly, the model demonstrates the importance of selecting diagnostically pure groups in research studies in this area, rather than heterogeneous groups of "dissociative disorder" patients (or individuals scoring high on the DES in non-clinical studies). Further evidence for the model could, however, be obtained from cluster analytic studies using mixed diagnostic groups and multiple measures of detachment and compartmentalization. In addition, further studies investigating the mechanisms of detachment and compartmentalization, using cognitive, neurophysiological and neuroimaging methods are urgently required.

Clinically, the model indicates that a "one size fits all" approach to treatment is invalid and highlights the importance of developing idiosyncratic formulations of dissociative disorder patients, based on an understanding of the specific psychological mechanisms of the problem in question. Recent evidence suggests that CBT using an adapted anxiety-disorder model is an effective treatment for pathological detachment (Hunter, Baker, Phillips, Sierra & David, 2005). Other forms of treatment may be more appropriate for pathological compartmentalization (for discussion see Holmes et al., 2005). Finally, the model questions the unqualified use of the term "dissociation" and emphasises the need to be much more specific about the kinds of phenomena that are being referred to when we use the label.

NOTES

1. Or, strictly speaking, *desagrégation*, which was subsequently translated into its English form.

2. This paper distinguishes between "symptoms" and "experiences." Both of these may be regarded as consciously identifiable subjective events; the assumption here is that only the former is associated with some kind of pathological process. The term "phenomena" is used as a collective label for both symptoms and experiences.

3. Amnesia is also identified as a symptom of peri-traumatic dissociation in ASD. In the Holmes et al. (2005) model, amnesia is a non-specific symptom that can be associated with either detachment or compartmentalization.

4. The SAS is comparable to the supervisory attentional system in the Norman and Shallice (1986) model.

5. The on-line generation of inhibitory programs by the SAS may play an important role in hypnotic and post-hypnotic amnesias (see Brown & Oakley, 2004).

6. The degree to which different working selves would have access to memories related to other selves would presumably also reflect the degree to which the goal hierarchies were in conflict.

REFERENCES

Allen, J. G. (2001). *Traumatic relationships and serious mental disorders.* New York, NY: John Wiley and Sons.

Allen, J. G., Console, D. A., & Lewis, L. (1999). Dissociative detachment and memory impairment: Reversible amnesia or encoding failure. *Comprehensive Psychiatry, 40,* 160-171.

American Psychiatric Association. (1994). *Diagnostic and Statistical Manual of Mental Disorders (4th ed.).* Washington, DC: Author.

Baker, D., Hunter, E., Lawrence, E., Medford, N., Patel, M., Senior, C., et al. (2003). Depersonalisation disorder: Clinical features of 204 cases. *British Journal of Psychiatry, 182,* 428-433.

Bernstein, E., & Putnam, F. W. (1986). Development, reliability and validity of a dissociation scale. *Journal of Nervous and Mental Disease, 174,* 727-735.

Blakemore, S-J., Wolpert, D.M., & Frith, C. D. (2002). Abnormalities in the awareness of action. *Trends in Cognitive Sciences, 6,* 237-242.

Blakemore, S-J., Oakley, D. A., & Frith, C. D. (2003). Delusions of alien control in the normal brain. *Neuropsychologia, 41,* 1058-67.

Brown, R. J. (2002a). The cognitive psychology of dissociative states. *Cognitive Neuropsychiatry, 7,* 221-235.

Brown, R. J. (2002b). Epilepsy, dissociation and nonepileptic seizures. In M. R. Trimble, & B. Schmitz (Eds.), *The neuropsychiatry of epilepsy* (pp. 189-209). Cambridge, UK: Cambridge University Press.

Brown, R. J. (2004). The psychological mechanisms of medically unexplained symptoms: An integrative conceptual model. *Psychological Bulletin, 130,* 793-812.

Brown, R. J., & Oakley, D. A. (2004). An integrative cognitive model of hypnosis and high hypnotisability. In M. Heap, R. J. Brown, & D. A. Oakley (Eds.), *The highly hypnotizable person: Theoretical, experimental and clinical issues* (pp. 152-186). London: Brunner-Routledge.

Butler, L. D., Duran, E. E., Jasiukaitis, P., Koopman, C., & Spiegel, D. (1996). Hypnotizability and traumatic experience: A diathesis-stress model of dissociative symptomatology. *American Journal of Psychiatry, 153,* 42-63.

Cardeña, E. (1994). The domain of dissociation. In S. J. Lynn, & J. W. Rhue (Eds.), *Dissociation: Clinical and Theoretical Perspectives* (pp. 15-31). New York, NY, USA: The Guilford Press.

Cassano, G. B., Petracca, A., Perugi, G., Toni, C., Tundo, A., & Roth, M. (1989). Derealization and panic attacks: Evaluation on 150 patients with panic disorder/agoraphobia. *Comprehensive Psychiatry, 30,* 5-12.

Conway, M. A. (2005). Memory and the self. *Journal of Memory and Language, 53,* 594-628.

Conway, M. A., & Pleydell-Pearce, C. W. (2000). The construction of autobiographical memories in the self-memory system. *Psychological Review, 107,* 261-288.

Dell, P. F. (2006). The multidimensional inventory of dissociation (MID): A comprehensive measure of pathological dissociation. *Journal of Trauma & Dissociation, 7*(2), 77-106.

Frankel, F. H. (1994). Dissociation in hysteria and hypnosis: A concept aggrandized. In S. J. Lynn & J. W. Rhue (Eds.), *Dissociation: Clinical and Theoretical Perspectives* (pp. 80-93). New York, NY, USA: The Guilford Press.

Hilgard, E. R. (1977). *Divided consciousness: Multiple controls in human thought and actions.* New York: Wiley.

Holmes, E., Brown, R. J., Mansell, W., Fearon, R. P, Hunter, E., Frasquilho, F., & Oakley, D. A. (2005). Are there two qualitatively distinct forms of dissociation? A review and some clinical implications. *Clinical Psychology Review, 25,* 1-23.

Hunter, E. C. M., Phillips, M. L., Chalder, T., Sierra, M., & David, A. S. (2003). Depersonalization disorder: A cognitive behavioural conceptualisation. *Behaviour Research and Therapy, 41,* 1451-1467.

Hunter, E. C. M., Baker, D., Phillips, M. L., Sierra, M., & David, A. S. (2005). Cognitive-behaviour therapy for depersonalisation disorder: An open study. *Behaviour Research and Therapy, 43,* 1121-1130.

Hunter, E. C. M., Sierra, M., & David, A. S. (2004). The epidemiology of depersonalisation and derealisation: A systematic review. *Social Psychiatry and Psychiatric Epidemiology, 39,* 9-18.

Jahanshahi, M., & Frith, C. D. (1998). Willed action and its impairments. *Cognitive Neuropsychology, 15,* 483-533.

Johnson, M. K., & Raye, C. L. (1981). Reality monitoring. *Psychological Review, 88,* 67-85.

Kihlstrom, J. F. (1992). Dissociative and conversion disorders. In D. J. Stein, & J. E. Young (Eds.), *Cognitive science and clinical disorders* (pp. 247-270). San Diego, CA7 Academic Press.

Kihlstrom, J. F. (1994). One hundred years of hysteria. In S. J. Lynn, & J. W. Rhue (Eds.), *Dissociation: Clinical and theoretical perspectives* (pp. 365-394). New York: Guilford Press.

Kirsch, I., & Lynn, S. J. (1997). Hypnotic involuntariness and the automaticity of everyday life. *American Journal of Clinical Hypnosis, 40,* 329-348.

Kosslyn, S. M. (1996). *Image and brain.* Cambridge, MA: MIT Press.

Kuyk, J., Spinhoven, P., & Van Dyck, R. (1999). Hypnotic recall: A positive criterion in the differential diagnosis between epileptic and pseudoepileptic seizures. *Epilepsia, 40,* 485-491.

Lambert, M. V., Sierra, M., Phillips, M. L., & David, A. S. (2002). The spectrum of organic depersonalization: A review plus four new cases. *Journal of Neuropsychiatry & Clinical Neurosciences, 14,* 141-154.

Logan, G. D. (1988). Toward an instance theory of automatization. *Psychological Review, 95,* 492-527.

Marcel, A. J. (1983). Conscious and unconscious perception: An approach to the relations between phenomenal experience and perceptual processes. *Cognitive Psychology, 15,* 238-300.

Marshall, R. D., Schneier, F. R., Lin, S., Simpson, H. B., Vermes, D., & Leibowitz, M. (2000). Childhood trauma and dissociative symptoms in panic disorder. *American Journal of Psychiatry, 157,* 451-453.

Nijenhuis, E. R. S., Spinhoven, P., Van Dyck, R., Van der Hart, O., & Vanderlinden, J. (1996). The development and the psychometric characteristics of the Somatoform Dissociation Questionnaire (SDQ-20). *Journal of Nervous and Mental Disease, 184,* 688-694.

Nijenhuis, E. R. S. (2004). *Somatoform dissociation.* New York: Norton.

Nijenhuis, E.R.S., Van der Hart, O., & Steele, K. (2004). Trauma-related structural dissociation of the personality. Trauma Information Pages website, January 2004: http://www.trauma-pages.com/nijenhuis-2004.htm

Norman, D. A., & Shallice, T. (1986). Attention to action: Willed and automatic control of behavior. In R. J. Davidson, G. E. Schwartz, & D. Shapiro (Eds.), *Consciousness and self-regulation: Vol. 4. Advances in research and theory* (pp. 1-18). New York: Plenum Press.

Noyes, R., & Kletti, R. (1977). Depersonalization in response to life-threatening danger. *Comprehensive Psychiatry, 8,* 375-384.

Oakley, D. A. (1999a). Hypnosis and conversion hysteria: A unifying model. *Cognitive Neuropsychiatry, 4,* 243-265.

Oakley, D. A. (1999b). Hypnosis and consciousness: A structural model. *Contemporary Hypnosis, 16,* 215-223.

Phillips, M. L., Medford, N., Senior, C., Bullmore, E. T., Brammer, M. J., Andrew, C., et al. (2001). Depersonalization disorder: thinking without feeling. Psychiatry Research. *Neuroimaging, 108,* 145-160.

Putnam, F. W. (1997). Dissociation in children and adolescents: A developmental perspective. New York: The Guilford Press.

Saxe, G. N., Van der Kolk, B. A., Berkowitz, R., Chinman, G. et al. (1993). Dissociative disorders in psychiatric inpatients. *American Journal of Psychiatry, 150,* 1037-1042.

Sierra, M., & Berrios, G. E. (1998). Depersonalization: Neurobiological perspectives. *Biological Psychiatry, 44,* 898-908.

Sierra, M., & Berrios, G. E. (2001). The phenomenological stability of depersonalization: Comparing the old with the new. *Journal of Nervous and Mental Disease, 189,* 629-636.

Sierra, M., Senior, C., Dalton, J., McDonough, M., Bond, A., Phillips, M. L., et al. (2002). Autonomic response in depersonalization disorder. *Archives of General Psychiatry, 59,* 833-838.

Simeon, D., Gross, S., Guralnik, O., Stein, D. J., Schmeidler, J., & Hollander, E. (1997). Feeling unreal: 30 cases of DSM-III-R Depersonalization Disorder. *American Journal of Psychiatry, 154,* 1107-1113.

Sloman, S. A. (1996). The empirical case for two systems of reasoning. *Psychological Bulletin, 119,* 3-22.

Steinberg, M. (1994). *Structured clinical interview for DSM-IV dissociative disorders (SCID-D), revised.* Washington, DC: American Psychiatric Press.

Sterlini, G. L., & Bryant, R. A. (2002). Hyperarousal and dissociation: A study of novice skydivers. *Behaviour Research and Therapy, 40,* 431-437.

Van der Hart, O. & Dorahy, M. J. (in press). Dissociation: History of a concept. In P. F. Dell & J. O'Neill (Eds.), *Dissociation and the dissociative disorders: DSM-V and beyond.* Chicago: International Society for the Study of Dissociation.

Van der Hart, O., Nijenhuis, E., Steele, K., & Brown, D. (2004). Trauma-related dissociation: Conceptual clarity lost and found. *Australian and New Zealand Journal of Psychiatry, 38,* 906-914.

Van der Kolk, B. A., & Fisler, R. (1995). Dissociation and the fragmentary nature of traumatic memories: Overview and exploratory study. *Journal of Traumatic Stress, 8,* 505-525.

van Ijzendoorn, M.H. & Schuengel, C. (1996). The measurement of dissociation in normal and clinical populations: Meta-analytic validation of the Dissociative Experiences Scale (DES). *Clinical Psychology Review, 16,* 365-382.

Velmans, M. (2000). *Understanding consciousness.* London: Routledge.

World Health Organization. (1992). The ICD-10 classification of mental and behavioural disorders: Clinical descriptions and diagnostic guidelines. Geneva, Switzerland: Author.

doi:10.1300/J229v07n04_02

The Dissociative Processing Style: A Cognitive Organization Activated by Perceived or Actual Threat in Clinical Dissociators

Martin J. Dorahy, PhD

SUMMARY. This paper proposes a cognitive organization that operates during times of perceived or actual threat in individuals with dissociative psychopathology. This organization, referred to as the dissociative processing style (DPS), serves as a threat monitoring system. It is characterized by (1) a shift from selective attention processing to multiple streams of information processing, (2) weakened cognitive inhibitory functioning which allows these streams to be operational and (3) the directing of awareness towards some and away from other information streams. Whilst DPS activation has the potential for adaptive and protective functions, it also heightens the likelihood of dissociative

Martin J. Dorahy is affiliated with the Trauma Resource Centre, North & West Belfast HSS Trust, and the School of Psychology, The Queen's University of Belfast, Northern Ireland.

Address correspondence to: Martin J. Dorahy, School of Psychology, David Keir Building, The Queen's University of Belfast, Belfast, BT9 5BP, Northern Ireland (E-mail: m.dorahy@qub.ac.uk).

The author would like to thanks Lisa Butler, PhD, Anne DePrince, PhD, Rafaële Huntjens, PhD, and 3 anonymous reviewers for their valuable comments on this manuscript.

[Haworth co-indexing entry note]: "The Dissociative Processing Style: A Cognitive Organization Activated by Perceived or Actual Threat in Clinical Dissociators." Dorahy, Martin J. Co-published simultaneously in *Journal of Trauma & Dissociation* (The Haworth Medical Press, an imprint of The Haworth Press, Inc.) Vol. 7, No. 4, 2006, pp. 29-53; and: *Exploring Dissociation: Definitions, Development and Cognitive Correlates* (ed: Anne P. DePrince, and Lisa DeMarni Cromer) The Haworth Medical Press, an imprint of The Haworth Press, Inc., 2006, pp. 29-53. Single or multiple copies of this article are available for a fee from The Haworth Document Delivery Service [1-800-HAWORTH, 9:00 a.m. - 5:00 p.m. (EST). E-mail address: docdelivery@haworthpress.com].

symptom experience and dissociation itself. Dissociation is understood as a failure to integrate encoded information from multiple input streams. The DPS is argued to be activated by top-down processes which signal danger, such as the appraisal of contextual cues. A clinical example is used to highlight the characteristics of the DPS. doi:10.1300/J229v07n04_03

[Article copies available for a fee from The Haworth Document Delivery Service: 1-800-HAWORTH. E-mail address: <docdelivery@haworthpress.com> Website: <http://www.HaworthPress.com> © 2006 by The Haworth Press, Inc. All rights reserved.]

KEYWORDS. Dissociative processing style, dissociation, cognition

The term dissociation has been used to denote (1) symptoms or phenomena (e.g., depersonalization; amnesia; daydreaming), (2) a process (i.e., breakdown in integrated functioning), with a corollary being defense,[1] and (3) a structural organization of the personality (e.g., a personality organization characterized by different degrees of division in typically integrated psychobiological action systems; Van der Hart, Nijenhuis & Steele, 2006), which may underlie various psychiatric conditions (Brenner, 2001; Chu, 1998; Van der Hart et al., 2006). These different uses of the term, and the more contemporary focus on phenomenology, have lead to concern that the word dissociation creates confusion and lacks specificity (e.g., Brown, this volume; Holmes et al., 2005; Van der Hart et al., 2006). Some have addressed this problem by limiting the specific symptoms that should be described as dissociation (e.g., Brown, this volume; Holmes et al., 2005). Others advocate restricting the term to its structural usage, indicating that dissociative symptoms are then defined as those phenomena that manifest directly from structural dissociation (i.e., the personality organization), and dissociation as a process is limited to failed integration of the personality (Van der Hart et al. 2006; see Dorahy & Van der Hart, in press).

Focusing on dissociation as a process, the current paper proposes a style of processing in clinical dissociators that has become a learned procedural skill and psychological strategy for dealing with perceived or actual threat from an internal and/or external source. A cognitive organization called the dissociative processing style (DPS),[2] activated in clinical dissociators in response to top-down information predicting potential threat or situations evoking heightened fear is proposed and explicated. DPS activation increases the likelihood of dissociation, which is understood as a failure to integrate *encoded* information from multiple input streams that without the process of dissociation would be brought together.[3] Therefore the process of dissociation in this paper relates to the failure to integrate encoded elements of an experience, rather than the failure to integrate psychobiological structures.[4] Dissociative encoding (i.e., the process of dissociation) is (1) a possible outcome of DPS activation and (2) the birthplace of dissociative symptoms such as partial amnesia, and visual and olfactory intrusions (see Kennedy et al., 2004, stage 1 dissociation). DPS activation is also argued to heighten the possibility of experiencing dissociative symptoms, especially of an intrusive type. This processing style represents a specific information processing type characterized by (1) a shift from selective attention processing to multiple streams of information processing, (2) weakened cognitive inhibitory functioning which allows these streams to be operational and (3) the directing of awareness towards some and away from other processing streams. These three components are not dissociation but characterize the DPS.

In this paper attention and conscious awareness are viewed as related constructs, with attention allowing an event or set of stimuli to be focused upon, and conscious awareness allowing the selected stimuli to be consciously experienced (Baars, 1997). The use of the term 'dissociative' in the proposed processing style reflects that this cognitive organization is present in individuals with dissociative pathology, rather than requiring that dissociation is an inevitable outcome when this processing style is activated. The formulation outlined here emphasizes information processing during moments of heightened anxiety in clinical dissociators (i.e., individuals in which dissociation is the central pathological mechanism).

DISSOCIATION AND THE DISSOCIATIVE PROCESSING STYLE: SETTING THE SCENE

As well as drawing on experimental cognitive studies of attentional functioning and information processing in dissociative disorders, this paper makes use of cognitive studies in (1) the non-clinical dissociation literature and (2) the literature on anxiety. Results from studies of cognitive functioning in non-clinical dissociators are less clouded by excessive anxiety, medication, or psychopathology (De Ruiter et al., this volume).[5] The anxiety literature is of importance because of the links between anxiety and dissociation (e.g., Gershuny, Cloitre, & Otto,

2003). Anxiety may be one of the central affective experiences that cues the dissociative processing style in those with this capability.

Dissociation and Memory

Dissociation is inextricably linked to memory encoding, consolidation and storage (Kihlstrom, 1987). The terms 'dissociation' and therefore by implication 'integration' can only relate to encoded information (Van der Hart et al., 2006). Individuals who reflexively shift attention away from encoding an event have not utilized or experienced dissociation. Whilst encoding, consolidation and storage are prerequisites for dissociation, dissociation also requires a *failure to integratively* encode, consolidate and store processed information (Van der Hart et al., 2006). Despite these memory processes being central (because without them dissociation is not possible), the assessment of dissociation and often its clinical manifestations (e.g., amnesia, flashbacks) are apparent through retrieval processes (i.e., the absence of retrieval in amnesia, the presence of non-volitional retrieval in flashbacks). Allen, Console and Lewis (1999) have further articulated the useful distinction between reversible and irreversible amnesia (see Brown, this volume; Holmes et al., 2005, for related discussions). Dissociative detachment (i.e., depersonalization and derealization; irreversible amnesia) during information processing involves to a greater or lesser extent a failure to elaboratively encode, consolidate and store memory. Allen et al. (1999) suggest that detachment is a form of dissociation. The current paper takes the view that detachment which blocks encoding is *associated with* dissociation, rather than *being* dissociation. Dissociation relates to the internal failure to integrate encoded sensory and psychobiological representations, not a failure to encode external, environmental stimuli (e.g., a road sign during highway hypnosis).

DISSOCIATION, INFORMATION PROCESSING, AND ANXIETY

Particularly since the renaissance of interest from the early 1970s, dissociation has been viewed as an innate non-pathological capacity (e.g., Butler, 2006; Ludwig, 1983) with a significant genetic loading (e.g., Becker-Blease et al., 2004). De Ruiter et al. (this volume), among others (e.g., Freyd, Martorello, Alvarado, Hayes & Christman, 1998), argue that because dissociation is an innate, dispositional variable, not reliant on environmental factors (e.g., trauma) for it (non-clinical) expression, dissociation will be related to basic cognitive functions.

Basic Cognitive Functioning and Dissociation

The most well-known experimental paradigm for assessing basic cognitive processes, such as the capturing of automatic, preattentive and attentive resources is the Stroop task (Stroop, 1935). In its most popular guise, participants are required to ignore the semantic meaning of a word and respond to its physical characteristics. In the crucial, incongruent trial the irrelevant semantic information conflicts directly with the target physical information (e.g., the word RED printed in green ink). The less processing resources are drawn to the irrelevant component the better task performance (which is measured in terms of speed or accuracy). Both Freyd et al. (1998) and DePrince and Freyd (1999) found greater interference in high non-clinical dissociators on the standard stroop task (i.e., naming ink color of colored words). The greater semantic processing of irrelevant color words in high dissociators may be derived from their heightened attentional and working memory capacities, which includes greater working memory span and efficiency, and elaborative processing (De Ruiter, Phaf, Elzinga, & Van Dyck, 2004; De Ruiter, Phaf, Veltman, Kok, & Van Dyck, 2003; Veltman et al., 2004). Greater elaborative processing of incoming information in high dissociators (Veltman et al., 2004; see also Elzinga et al., 2000, study 1; De Ruiter et al., this volume) may lead to enhanced information processing of even task irrelevant word meaning, producing increased stroop interference. The findings from these studies suggest that dissociation, as measured by experiential phenomena, is an adaptive capacity (DePrince & Freyd, 2001; DeRuiter et al., 2004, this volume) related to greater (1) attentional ability, (2) working memory functioning and capacity, and (3) memory encoding. *These cognitive features of high dissociators, as well as possibly producing stroop interference, also provide the necessary basic functional building blocks for the development of the dissociative processing style.*

Emotional Stroop, Selective Attention and Dissociation

The so-called emotional stroop task has been developed to examine the impact of irrelevant, though personally significant stimuli on information processing. Color words are replaced by non-color words or stimuli emotionally linked and relevant to the individual's distress

(Matthews & Harley, 1996). The emotional stroop task produces robust findings in anxious, non-clinical individuals and especially in mood and anxiety disorders (Matthews & Harley, 1996; William, Mathews & MacLeod, 1996): An attentional bias (i.e., the capturing of preattentional/attentional resources by the irrelevant but personally significant stimulus and resultant slowing of color naming) is present for word stimulus directly related to the core theme of psychopathology (e.g., Mathews & MacLeod, 1985; McNally, Kaspi, Reimann, & Zeitlin, 1990; Watts, McKenna, Sharrock, & Trezise, 1986). Emotional stroop interference rests on words being central to the individual's current concerns and negative/threatening (Williams et al., 1996). Simeon (personal communication, March, 2006) demonstrated a trend towards emotional stroop interference in individuals with depersonalization disorder using words associated with the experience of depersonalization (e.g., 'foggy,' 'unreal,' 'spacey'; Simeon, Knutelska, Putnam, Schmeidler & Smith, 2005). This tentatively indicates that individuals with pathological dissociation fear dissociative experiences, and consequently have processing resources drawn to words associated with them.

In more complex dissociative disorders, the capturing of automatic processes by threat cues may be dependent on the nature of the dissociative part of the personality assessed. In a DID sample Hermans et al. (2006) found support for the view that trauma-avoidant identities evade the processing of threat stimuli at an automatic level, while trauma-fixated identities are drawn towards them. It is argued here that following DPS activation automatic processes are primed towards threat stimuli (like trauma-fixated identities), but the activation of multiple stream of processing provides the potential for avoidance (like trauma-avoidant identities) of threat streams.

Divided Attention and Multiple Information Processing Streams

Theoretical conjecture and empirical findings show high dissociators are particularly gifted at, and operate cognitively more effectively when, dividing their attention and utilizing multiple streams of information processing (DePrince & Freyd, 1999; Freyd, 1996; Simeon et al., 2005). This evokes questions regarding the relationship between encoding and the operation of multiple processing streams. Using a recall task of stroop words, Simeon et al. (2005) found evidence that their depersonalization disorder group failed to encode threat stimuli in the divided attention task, at least to the level available for free recall. Using a recognition task, DePrince and Freyd (2004) found solid indications that divided attention in high dissociators may lead to the complete failure to encode threatening stimuli.

The findings of DePrince and Freyd (2004) and Simeon et al. (2005) suggests that in an effort to avoid threat stimuli divided attention may serve a protective function by reducing the likelihood that such stimuli are encoded. Encoding failures are without doubt a feature of dissociative disorders (e.g., Allen et al., 1999). Yet, encoding failure does not explain or account for dissociation. For example, data indicates that clinical dissociators have trouble stopping the encoding of threat stimuli (Elzinga, Phaf, Ardon, & Van Dyck, 2003). Moreover, dissociation is related to the encoding of threat information processed outside awareness. This is suggested by the widespread observation that traumatic information is often retrieved for the first time long after encoding (e.g., sometimes in therapy), which on account of the individual reporting no prior memory of it, may have been encoded outside awareness. Based on empirical work, Hilgard (see 1986 for review) proposed a model where semi-independent subordinate cognitive structures, which support multiple streams of processing, can operate outside conscious awareness and effectively encode information later available for explicit retrieval.[6] Thus, memory encoding can occur during the operation of multiple streams of processing and can occur for information streams processed outside awareness. Encoding failure may be a cognitive feature of clinical dissociators, but the DPS is characterized by the encoding of information from multiple stream of information processing. Dissociation, the final, though not inevitable, outcome of DPS activation, is the failure to integrate these multiple encoded streams.

A divided attention strategy may be particularly beneficial and effective when processing threat information as awareness of this information can be reduced if divided attention strategies are utilized and threat is processed but ignored (DePrince & Freyd, 2001; Simeon et al., 2005). In high non-clinical dissociators, De Ruiter et al. (2003) found that detection and response to target stimuli in a letter detection task was facilitated in threat words. This suggests the threat valence of the words captured attention in high dissociators, but rather than impacting detrimentally on target responding, actually assisted it (arguably Hermans et al.'s findings in the trauma-avoidant identities display a similar phenomenon). De Ruiter et al. (2003) suggested that high dissociators had better divided attention abilities (i.e., they could process irrelevant stimuli with an absence of detrimental effect to relevant stimuli responding) which may be particularly evident when confronted with affective stimuli.

These findings indicate that *during times of divided attention processing high dissociators are able to shift awareness away from the information processing stream that contains affective stimuli and onto the stream that contains the non-affective stimuli which requires a response.*[7] Such a conclusion is merited by the high dissociators capacity to efficiently respond to non-affective target stimuli in the affective stimulus pieces. This finding suggests that high dissociators engage in avoidance of threat processing streams when non-threatening streams are also being processed. Yet, other work has shown that when the *target* stimulus is threatening and divided attention cannot be used to avoid it, high dissociator participants respond slower (Waller, Quinton & Watson, 1995).

Avoidance and the DPS

Several studies have reported that individuals with a high dissociative propensity attempt to avoid the processing of threatening information (DePrince & Freyd, 2004; Foa & Hearst-Ikeda, 1996; Waller et al., 1995). Yet, other studies of dissociation (e.g., De Ruiter et al., 2003) and the anxiety literature suggest that feared stimuli attract preattentive/ attentive operations, at least at the very early stages of processing. So dissociative individuals should in the first instance shunt automatic resources towards, rather than away from, threat. The attentional avoidance of threat information comes following early detection of threat in those with a dissociative processing style, where attention is protectively directed towards information processing streams that are emotionally unthreatening or innocuous, such as the colour of the bedroom walls for a girl being sexually abused, or the *location* of cars and bodies, and the task at hand for Mr. X (See 'Mr. X' below).

The redirection of awareness away from threat streams is a learned, trial and error process, that develops like trauma-phobias in clinical dissociators (Steele, Van der Hart & Nijenhuis, 2005; Van der Hart et al., 2006). With ongoing noxious events the dissociative individual learns to direction awareness away from emotionally painful streams and onto less threatening details whilst experiencing a traumatic event. Freyd (1996), among others (e.g., De Ruiter et al., 2003; Elzinga et al., 2000), has suggested that individuals with high dissociative capacities use their divided attention skills to keep stored traumatic memories out of awareness by focusing on other information streams so as to reduce trauma retrieval. As well as being used to lessen the *retrieval* of trauma, the same capacity too avoid threat may be present during *encoding* (see Cloitre, 1992, for further discussion). Consequently awareness is directed towards non-threatening and away from threatening streams of information during processing and encoding, not just following memory storage or as a way to regulate traumatic memory retrieval.

The redirection of awareness away from information streams processing threatening information is not dissociation (i.e, failure to integrate encoded information), but may be a characteristic of the dissociative processing style. This learned pattern within the dissociative processing style shifts awareness onto information streams containing non-emotive contents or tasks of everyday life, as such it serves a protective purpose. When the DPS operates optimally to protect the individual, awareness is automatically directed away from threat streams. Therefore the protective value of this aspect of the DPS is related to the degree to which awareness is shunted away from threat streams at the time of processing. Yet, even with a less protective action (i.e., awareness on some or all streams containing threat material) dissociation could still take place. As multiple streams of processing implies a failure to be aware of them all (Cloitre, 1992), non-emotive aspects may be processed outside awareness while the traumatic content of the event may be in focal awareness. Such a scenario is evident clinically when individuals become aware for the first time of non-threatening aspects of a traumatic event in therapy (e.g., the location of the growing crowd of onlookers in the case of Mr. X, below).

The current model suggests that dissociation and the directing of conscious awareness onto specific streams of processing are two separate components associated with the DPS. Each of these components has the capacity to offer protection against painful stimuli, but at different stages within the system. When the DPS is characterized by the avoidance of threat streams during encoding, protection is offered against the full emotional, cognitive and existential force of the event. Alternatively, dissociation (failure to integrate the encoded content of multiple information streams) may demonstrate protective capabilities most noticeable during retrieval. For example, an individual could be aware of both non-traumatic and traumatic details of an event during encoding (i.e., if awareness is not directed away from streams with traumatic content), but could have recall failure for the traumatic information at a later point if retrieval processes become focused on other stored aspects of the event (which due to the failure to integrate the separate streams of information representing all encoded details of the event are disassociated from the threat material).

Notably, dissociation and the DPS from the current perspective are not defensive in the same way as psychodynamic ego defenses. The phylogenetic purpose of the ego-defenses is psychic defense, and they are active strategies for reducing psychological tension and psychic threat (Freud, 1926). Shifting awareness away from threat streams is a learned strategy that may, but does not necessarily, characterize the DPS. Therefore, the DPS may, but does not necessarily, have a protective function of threat avoidance. Of course, the psychological motivation for the development of a dissociative processing style in the first instance requires attention at a latter point and may be motivated by protective aspirations. Dissociation within the dissociative processing style undoubtedly has the capacity to serve a protective functioning. However, further theoretical and empirical work is required to determine if this is the primary function of failed integration or if the failure to integrate multiple encoded streams of information during heightened stress is primarily the result of the brain's inability to bind the various psychobiological (including cognitive), experiential and environmental aspects, with the byproduct being protective.

To summarize thus far, the current paper argues that clinical dissociators have a psychological structure which when activated by perceived or actual threat leads to a dissociative processing style for cognitively dealing with environmental and psychosomatic representations. This DPS is characterized by the activation of multiple streams of information processing and the shifting of awareness away from some and onto other streams during processing. Dissociation, which may be one outcome of the DPS, is the failure to integrate the encoded material from separate processing streams. Encoding failure brought about by avoidance strategies may be common in individuals with heightened dissociative symptoms, but is not associated directly with dissociation. Avoidance in the DPS relates to the shifting of awareness from threat streams.

Cognitive Inhibition

With high dissociators having the best chance of keeping threatening information from awareness when attention can be divided (DePrince & Freyd, 2001), the greatest protective value from threat during information processing is offered when multiple streams of processing are operational. Recent studies of cognitive inhibition offer one explanation for how this may be achieved in individuals with heightened levels of dissociative experience. Selection of target stimuli in the cognitive system is a dual opponent process: facilitation of information to be attended to, and active inhibition of information competing for attention but peripheral to target selection (Fox, 1995; Neill, 1977; Tipper & Cranston, 1985). Thus cognitive inhibition is believed to be central to selective attention and working memory functioning (e.g., Hasher & Zacks, 1988).

Bjorklund and Harnishfeger (1995) maintain that cognitive inhibition is a means of regulating conscious content and limiting attentional processes to those aspects most pertinent to dealing with current tasks. They note that cognitive inhibition refers to several related processes, including (1) the capacity to withhold distracting information from ongoing processing, (2) the clearing from working memory of currently selected but irrelevant information, and (3) the ability to withhold from conscious awareness previously selected information. Giesbrecht, Merckelbach, Geraerts and Smeets (2004) found that student participants with higher scores on the DES amnesia subscale (but not the DES-absorption or depersonalization/derealization subscales) and the DES-T demonstrated reduced inhibitory capacity in clearing working memory of previously selected material and withholding previously activated information. They suggested their results indicated a link between inhibitory failures and pathological dissociation, especially that related to memory functioning.

Initial studies with high non-clinical and pathologically anxious individuals have shown weakened inhibition for threat-related material (Amir, Coles & Foa, 2002; Wood, Mathews & Dalgleish, 2001). Studies of pathological dissociators indicate that cognitive inhibitory functioning is also related to the emotional context of the test environment. In conditions where individuals with DID were given the pre-assessment message that some presented stimuli would be threatening, or in experimental contexts where they reported elevated anxiety, cognitive inhibitory functioning was weakened (Dorahy, Irwin & Middleton, 2002; Dorahy, Middleton & Irwin, 2005). In contexts where DID participants were told that only single digit numbers (i.e., non-threatening stimuli) would be presented or where they reported a stable baseline level of anxiety, inhibitory functioning operated effectively (Dorahy, Irwin & Middleton, 2004; Dorahy, Middleton & Irwin, 2004). This influence of anxiety on inhibitory functioning in high dissociators was most clearly evident in a study in which DID, generalized anxiety disorder (GAD) and non-clinical control participants were assessed in neutral and threatening contexts manipulated by pre-assessment instruction and test stimuli (Dorahy, McCusker, Loewenstein, Colbert, & Mulholland, 2006). The DID sample demonstrated effective inhibition in the neutral, non-threatening context, like the control sample. However, in the threatening context, they showed weakened inhibitory functioning. This pattern was not present in the GAD sample. Both this and previous work suggest that the weakening of inhibitory functioning in threat contexts is a cognitive process related to dissociative capacity, rather than anxiety (Dorahy et al., 2006) or depression (Dorahy et al., 2005). *Thus, the dissociative processing style should be characterized by weakened inhibitory functioning as it becomes activated during times of heightened anxiety.*

Dorahy et al. (2006) have argued that reduced cognitive inhibition during situations of heightened anxiety may be adaptive for dissociative individuals. This is because of the role reduced inhibition plays in assisting the activation of multiple streams of information processing. With inhibitory processes operating effectively, selective attention is optimized by the withholding of superfluous environmental and psychosomatic representations. More information requires processing with weakened inhibition. High dissociators, with their capacity to function effectively with multiple streams of processing in operation (DePrince & Freyd, 2001; Hilgard, 1986, 1994), will be able to deal more efficiently with the greater demands created by weakened inhibition. Individuals without this capacity will be overwhelmed by the greater cognitive demands. Weakened inhibition therefore increases environmental and psychosomatic processing demands to allow the more efficient multiple stream of information processing in dissociative individuals during times of heightened anxiety. In other words, the extra information processing required when inhibition is weakened allows the operation of multiple streams in those with this ability (i.e., those characterized by increased dissociative phenomenology).

The DPS has adaptive potential for high dissociators in contexts of heightened arousal. Yet, the DPS is also argued to leave those who are capable of, and utilize, it open to (1) dissociation (i.e., dissociative encoding) and (2) intrusive dissociative symptoms (e.g., flashbacks, dissociative intrusions). Heightened probability of intrusive dissociative symptoms may be the direct result of weakened inhibition during DPS activation (Dorahy & Huntjens, in press). With weakened inhibition and more information processing streams operational during DPS activation, working memory is more likely to be intruded upon by top-down threat information from long-term memory. The re-experiencing of dissociatively stored information during DPS activation and weakened inhibition may be the result of associative learning cues, where either physical stimuli and/or the psychological context itself, triggers associated memories (Cloitre, 1992). The so-called dissociative or amnestic barriers, which may otherwise keep information compartmentalized, have been found to be more permeable than initially assumed (e.g., Huntjens et al., 2003). Turning to dissociation during DPS activation, the clinical case of Mr. X provides a clear example, and also highlights the proposed cognitive features of the DPS.

Mr. X

Mr. X was an emergency services worker in the Belfast area who had been exposed to not only the regular carnage that his job entailed but also the aftermath of numerous terrorist attacks associated with the Northern Irish 'Troubles.' On presentation at the clinic he reported numerous traumatic events in his occupational and personal history. However, one incident in particular continued to haunt him and lead to his early retirement from work. He described that his team was called to an accident, the details of which were conveyed en route over the radio and which gave some indication of the horrific scene that awaited them. On arrival Mr. X assessed the dangers along with the location of the vehicles and bodies involved. He also assumed coordination duty for his team, directed junior members, and commenced his own tasks. In describing the event during assessment he remembered clearly the location and state of the vehicles and bodies (particularly the graphic nature of the injuries), the tasks he fulfilled whilst at the accident scene, the directives he gave to his team and other personnel during the clean-up operation and the thoughts that were running through his mind regarding the victim's families being informed of their deaths. During the memory processing stage of treatment Mr. X became aware of several details of the accident which he must have encoded at the time but had no awareness of either then or since. These included the strong smell of burning blood and the location and size of the crowd of on-lookers.

The horrific nature of the accident scene, as described in the radio report on the way to the job, elicited feelings of anxiety. At a cognitive level weakened inhibition ensued and due to his heightened dissociative capacity multiple information processing streams became activated. Arriving at the scene these multiple streams of information processing were encoding and storing different aspects of environmental, sensory and psychosomatic/psychobiological representations. These included visual information (e.g., where bodies were in relation to other objects, like cars), olfactory stimuli (e.g., the smell of burning oil and blood). Moreover, at least one stream of processing which was taking in the key environmental variables required to assist declarative and procedural knowledge to allow him to coordinate others and efficiently do his own job as the lead emergency services worker at the scene. At the time of processing he was aware of (i.e., experiencing) highly distressing details of the event, and therefore DPS activation did not include complete avoidance of streams with trauma content (perhaps because the extent of traumatic representations all around him made this impossible). However, whether prompted by active avoidance or the hardware limitation of being unable to be aware of all processing streams, an olfactory stream encoded the smell of blood outside awareness.

Multiple streams of processing, with encoding of information outside awareness, along with dissociation,[8] are central to the fact that on presentation at the clinic many years after the event, Mr. X was unaware of the onlookers or the smell of burning blood (yet, he often reported being awoken by a strong smell which he could not identify). If Mr. X had a reduced capacity for multiple streams of processing and the processing of some of these streams outside awareness, lesser encoding of the various aspects and representations of the scene would have taken place (perhaps including the olfactory stream with burning blood). Hilgard (1994) makes a similar point when he states that individuals without the capacity to process one of several streams of information outside awareness will "fail to record and store in memory events not in focus" (p. 45). With reference to dissociation, if integration rather than dissociation had of occurred between these various information streams his memory of the event would have always included the fact he could smell burning blood.

ACTIVATION OF THE DISSOCIATIVE PROCESSING STYLE

The DPS effectively operates as a threat monitoring system engaged when in, or just prior to entering, anxiety provoking contexts and before threat stimuli are actually confronted. The Stroop literature in anxiety disorders will assist in further understanding DPS activation. Williams et al. (1996) suggested that emotional stroop interference results from mental representations of threat stimuli having (1) higher resting activation levels and (2) increased output responsiveness than neutral stimuli. Consequently, automatic processes immediately become attracted to stimuli whose mental representations are imbued with these qualities. Yet these qualities, which mark a mental representation as threatening, are not permanently bestowed on these representations, a strategic process is required to activate them. Matthews and Harley (1996) identified a threat monitoring unit which, when activated, primes automatic processes to stimuli deemed potentially threatening by the threat monitor, so that such stimuli attract resources at the earliest stage of processing. Thus emotional Stroop interference comes about when a controlled process (i.e., the threat monitoring unit) is activated, for example, by contextual factors such as a crowd of people in those with social phobia. This activation then heightens responsivity at the automatic level for stimuli related to the fear, which in turn leads to the greater automatic allocation of processing resources to threat stimuli when present (Fox, 1996; Matthews & Harley, 1996). This theory is consistent with Fox's (1996) findings that automatic processes were responsible for attentional bias to threat but the bias was only present when automatic processes were first primed by threat detection at the attentional level. In short, this suggests that automatic processes are not 'eternally vigilant' to feared stimuli, but require contextual, strategic, top-down information to prime or activate automatic processes to threat (Fox, 1996).

Building on these findings the Self-Regulatory Executive Function (S-REF) model was developed and outlines the interaction between 3 levels of control within the attention-memory system: automatic processes, controlled processes and long-term memory (e.g., Wells & Matthews, 1994, Matthews & Wells, 1999). A backward (top-down) feed operates so that long-term memory plays a pivotal role in controlled processes and controlled processes play a pivotal role, through mechanisms like priming, in automatic processing (e.g., threat monitoring which is an activity of controlled processes primes automatic processes to internal and external threat cues). Wells and Matthews specify a mode or unit of functioning called the S-REF. This mode of functioning is part of the controlled processing level and is primarily activated by top-down long-term memory processes. Activation of the S-REF includes monitoring for threat and as such primes automatic processes towards potential threat information, creating the selection bias evident in the emotional stroop (Matthews & Harley, 1996). Activation of the S-REF is required to switch automatic operations to biasedly detect and process stimuli deemed threatening.

The DPS has some analogous features with the S-REF. Firstly, the DPS is not always activated and therefore dissociative individuals are not always "on guard" cognitively. But when activated the DPS operates as a threat monitoring system. In the DPS this not only occurs through the priming of automatic processes to threat stimuli, but by weakened cognitive inhibition and multiple processing streams which principally allow faster threat detection (De Ruiter et al., 1993). Whilst DPS activation can come from the attentional detection of threat (i.e., perceiving actual threat), it typically comes from top-down cues which signal potential threat, like (1) the appraisal of contextual information[9] (e.g., "It's now dark, I'm in more danger"), (2) anticipated threat (e.g., "I'm out of the house and therefore I'm more vulnerable") or (3) external declarative information, such as experimental instructions that threat material will appear (see Figure 1).

DPS activation puts the dissociative individual into a state of psychological preparedness where reduced cognitive inhibition and the multiple processing streams allow more inputs from the potentially hostile environment to be taken in. This organization has the capacity to provide faster detection and response to threat stimuli, and in this sense is adaptive.[10] However, with a history of needing to (psychologically) escape the (physically and perhaps psychologically) inescapable (Freyd, 1996), dissociative individuals learn to evade threat streams (i.e., shift conscious awareness from these streams). This evasion of threat information speeds their response to non-threat streams if such is required (e.g., naming stroop ink colour), but retards their actions if a response is required to the threat stimuli (see Waller et al., 1995, for one of the few studies that thoroughly assessed this later hypothesis). Thus, while traumatized, high dissociators are argued here to have the psychological architecture to *detect* threat quickly (i.e., when the DPS is activated) their actually *response* to threat is impeded. An explanation for the faster detection of, but slower reaction to, threat cues requires investigation.

SOME IMPLICATIONS OF THE DPS

One therapeutic and two conceptual implications of the DPS will be briefly mentioned. First, as an overlearned procedural information processing strategy during times of heightened anxiety the DPS appears relatively automatized to dissociative individuals, who feel they automatically enter this state of psychological hypervigilance and processing. Yet in actual fact DPS activation is largely regulated by strategic/controlled processes, making it amendable to conscious/willed control. The fact that DPS activation increases the likelihood of dissociative encoding (i.e., dissociation) and dissociative symptom experience usually

FIGURE 1. Components of the DPS, and its strategic activation and automatic responsivity.

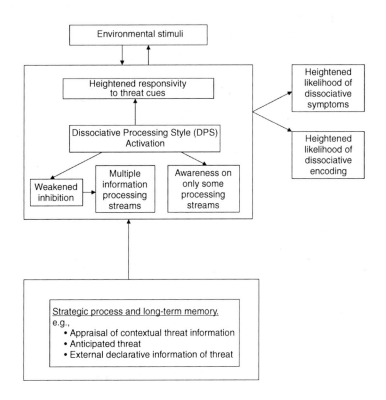

means its management and control is a central focus in the early stages of therapy. The therapeutic step of bringing DPS activation under conscious control may be assisted by an awareness in the client that this seemingly automatized processing style is largely driven by contextual (e.g., "other people are dangerous") and self-referenced (e.g., "I can't manage when I'm out of the house") appraisals. Managing DPS activation is central for affect tolerance work, with the ultimate goal being the capacity to experience increasingly greater levels of anxiety without DPS activation (and the potentially resultant dissociative encoding or dissociative symptom experience).

Second, Bromberg (1998) has noted the vigilance that often characterizes dissociative individuals and operates to allow them to feel they are prepared for threat when (not if) it comes. DPS activation may characterize the cognitive components of Bromberg's "dissociative vigilence" (p. 230). Particularly in more severe dissociative disorders the DPS may be activated nearly continuously on account of general appraisals of the world and other people being unsafe (e.g., Chu, 1998). Ongoing reactivity to treat cues reinforces appraisals regarding the dangerousness of contact with the world and other people, which maintains DPS activation when the individual is required to 'engage in life.'

Third, failure to attend to threat streams during processing may account for some episodes of revictimization (Butler, personal communication, April, 2006), which is so prevalent in those with dissociative disorders (e.g., Kluft, 1990). Processing threat information outside awareness may leave an individual oblivious to potential threat cues that would reshape their behavior (e.g., "this dark street looks dangerous, I'll walk a safer way").

FUTURE THEORETICAL TASKS

Several core issues require future attention. First, failure to encode information is common in dissociative disorders (e.g., Allen et al., 1999). This characteristic, so visible in the clinical setting, may be another outcome of DPS activation, but if so, how, and under what conditions does encoding and encoding failure occur outside awareness?

Second, links from the current proposal to structural models of dissociation (e.g., Van der Hart et al., 2006) are required. In complex dissociative disorders the activation of different dissociative structures may be associated with different processing streams. An individual with DID may fail to integrate encoded information because when the DPS is activated and threat stimuli are then confronted, the threat information (along with the bulk of the affect) may be encoded in a part of the personality fixated in threat. This encoding and knowledge of the actual stimulus itself may occur outside awareness because the stream in awareness is processing non-threat stimulus which is encoded into a part of the personality that is trauma-avoidant. Thus, as well as exploring the bottom-up aspects of these multiple streams (i.e., input information), future work must address their top-down aspects in light of structural models of dissociation.

Third, the nature of dissociative encoding itself requires attention. The processing of streams outside awareness may effect the quality of encoding (Kihlstrom, 1987). Freyd (1996) has suggested that information not consciously processed may not be stored as a declarative memory, but instead as a sensory or procedural memory trace. Thus if during traumatic experiences multiple streams of processing operate there may be some encoding but it may lack full elaboration (Ehlers & Clark, 2000), reducing its integrative potential. Recent studies in the non-clinical population have supported a link between dissociation and reduced elaboration (e.g., Holmes, Brewin & Hennessy, 2004, but compare Kindt & Van den Hout, 2003). A further possibility is that memory elaboration and perhaps integration of an experience could happen to a greater extent if encoding occurred in dissociative structures whose content was consistent with the experience being processed. In this case there may be less dissociative encoding of the separate aspects of the experience (even though this may still occur), and the dissociation would come from the integrative encoding into a structure which is itself disconnected from other psychobiological structures (Van der Hart et al., 2006). These explanations are not mutually exclusive as non-elaborated memories could, and most certainly are, encoded in dissociative structures.

Fourth, a further understanding is required of when activation of the DPS does and does not produce dissociative encoding. Dissociative encoding has been described here as a potential, rather than inevitable, outcome of DPS activation. This is on account of the possibility that during times of multiple streams of processing in contexts of heightened anxiety integration of encoded stimuli may occur. Determining when dissociative encoding occurs may be assisted by a greater knowledge of DPS operations when the individual shifts from a hypervigilant state of threat monitoring to actually being confronted with a threat stimulus or attacked.

CONCLUSION

This paper focused on the process of dissociation, with near exclusive attention on the proposed cognitive organization that operates in clinical dissociators during times of heightened anxiety and which may produce dissociation (i.e., dissociative encoding). Dissociation itself was not explored (e.g., the mechanisms of failed integration) but was understood as the failure to integrate or bind encoded representations (e.g., environmental stimuli) and internal features (e.g., affects, cognitions) from multiple streams of information processing. This failure to integrate encoded information (i.e., dissociation) is one possible outcome of the proposed DPS. Failure to encode information may also turn out to be an outcome of DPS activation, but this failure is not dissociation, regardless of whether active avoidance explains such phenomena.

The DPS outlined here is effectively a threat monitoring module engaged primarily by top-down activation and characterized by reduced cognitive inhibition, multiple information processing streams and non-awareness of the content of some of these processing streams. It has its foundation in the enhanced working memory and attentional capacities associated with heightened dissociative experience. The protective value of the DPS *during* processing comes from the degree to which awareness can be deviated from streams containing threat content. Future work may find that dissociative structures (e.g., dissociative identities) impinge on processing streams and avoidance or attraction to threat information may be influence by which dissociative structures are involved in processing at that moment. Activation of the DPS was argued to be associated not only with dissociation but also a heightened vulnerability to intrusive dissociative symptoms. The benefit of DPS activation for threat monitoring is offset by the increased likelihood of dissociation and dissociative symptom experience. Further explication of the DPS, and integration with clinical, theoretical and empirical advances in the understanding of dissociative disorders is required if this model offers some value.

NOTES

1. The issue of dissociation as a defense has alone been the focus of different viewpoints. For example, within the psychoanalytic literature dissociation is utilized in different ways, including as a defensive mechanism of the ego, as splitting of the ego or as the incomplete or partial integration ("unintegration," Winnicott, 1945) of very early emotional processes in infants (e.g., Brenner, 2001; Vaillant, 1992; Winnicott, 1945). Dissociation as defense is central to all these conceptualizations. Dissociation as a form of avoidance has been proffered by cognitive theorists to link the construct with its hypothesized affect management/defensive capacities (e.g., Foa & Hearst-Ikeda, 1996). Others have suggested that defensive aspects of dissociation are secondary, coming as a consequence, not a function, of dissociation (Janet, 1907; Van der Hart et al., 2006).

2. The term 'dissociative processing style' is derived from descriptions, largely in the non-clinical dissociation literature, of a dissociative style (De Ruiter, Elzinga & Phaf, this volume; Elzinga, De Beurs, Sergeant, Van Dyck, & Phaf, 2000), a dissociative defense style (Spiegel, 1986) or a dissociative coping style (Irwin, 1998).

3. This paper limits itself to dissociation in the information processing/memory domain. It does not address dissociation in other domains (e.g., conation).

4. The failure to integrate all encoded aspects of an experience (i.e., dissociation as defined in this paper) may be related to, but appears to operate at a level below and therefore could be distinct from, the relatively complete integration of encoded aspects of an experience which is assimilated into a dissociated psychobiological structure (e.g., 'a dissociative part of the personality,' Van der Hart et al., 2006).

5. Despite the possible benefits in drawing upon non-clinical cognitive studies of dissociation to inform cognitive functioning in clinical dissociators, this strategy may be limited by possible differences in non-clinical and clinical dissociation. Thus the proposed model relies upon empirical validation.

6. Janet (1907) also noted this phenomenon in hysteria.

7. Brown (2004) points out that traumatized individuals often shift attention onto bodily experiences during the processing of a traumatic event, keeping cognitive and affective components of the experience outside awareness.

8. Whilst encoding outside awareness and dissociation have been separated here, future work may identify the characteristics which determine when they are one and the same thing.

9. Cloitre (1992) has noted that experiencing sensory and perceptual cues reminiscent of prior threat are particularly powerful primers, and here would be argued to activate the DPS.

10. A heightened likelihood of dissociative encoding and dissociative symptom experience represent the maladaptive dimensions of the DPS.

REFERENCES

Allen, J. G., Console, D. A., & Lewis, L. (1999). Dissociative detachment and memory impairment: Reversible amnesia or encoding failure. *Comprehensive Pyschiatry*, *40*, 160-171.

Amir, N., Coles, M. E., & Foa, E. B. (2002). Automatic and strategic activation and inhibition of threat-relevant information in posttraumatic stress disorder. *Cognitive Therapy and Research*, *26*, 645-655.

Baars, B. J. (1997). Some essential differences between consciousness and attention, perception, and working memory. *Consciousness and Cognition*, *6*, 363-371.

Becker-Blease, K. A., Deater-Deckard, K., Eley, T., Freyd, J. F., Stevenson, J., & Plomin, R. (2004). A genetic analysis of individual differences in dissociative behaviors in childhood and adolescence. *Journal of Child Psychology and Psychiatry*, *45*, 522-532.

Bjorklund, D. F., & Harnishfeger, K. K. (1995). The evolution of inhibition mechanisms and their role in human cognition and behaviour. In F. N. Dempster & C. J. Brainerd (Eds.), *Interference and inhibition in cognition* (pp. 141-173). San Diego, CA: Academic Press.

Brenner, I. (2001). *Dissociation of trauma: Theory, phenomenology, and technique*. Madison, CT: International Universities Press.

Bromberg, P. M. (1998). *Standing in the spaces: Essays on clinical process, trauma and dissociation*. Hillsdale, NJ: The Analytic Press.

Brown, R. J. (2004). Psychological mechanisms of medically unexplained symptoms: An integrative conceptual model. *Psychological Bulletin, 130,* 793-812.

Butler, L. D. (2006). Normative dissociation. *Psychiatric Clinics of North America, 29,* 45-62.

Chu, J. A. (1998). *Rebuilding shattered lives: The responsible treatment of Complex Post-traumatic and Dissociative Disorders.* New York: John Wiley & Sons.

Cloitre, M. (1992). Avoidance of emotional processing: A cognitive science perspective. In D. J. Stein & J. E. Young (Eds.), *Cognitive science and clinical disorders* (pp. 19-41). San Diego, CA: Academic Press, Inc.

DePrince, A. P., & Freyd, J. J. (1999). Dissociation, attention and memory. *Psychological Science, 10,* 449-452.

DePrince, A. P., & Freyd, J. J. (2001). Memory and dissociative tendencies: The role of attentional context and word meaning in a directed forgetting task. *Journal of Trauma and Dissociation, 2,* 67-82.

DePrince, A. P., & Freyd, J.J. (2004). Forgetting trauma stimuli. *Psychological Science, 15,* 488-492.

De Ruiter, M. B., Phaf, R. H., Elzinga, B. M., & Van Dyck, R. (2004). Dissociative style and individual differences in verbal working memory span. *Consciousness and Cognition, 13,* 821-828.

De Ruiter, M. B., Phaf, R. H., Veltman, D. J., Kok, A., & Van Dyck, R. (2003). Attention as a characteristic of non-clinical dissociation: An event-related potential study. *NeuroImage, 19,* 376-390.

Dorahy, M. J., & Huntjens, R. J. C. (in press). Memory and attentional processes in Dissociative Identity Disorder: A review of the empirical literature. In E. Vermetten, M. J. Dorahy, & D. Spiegel (Eds.), *Traumatic dissociation: Neurobiology and treatment.* Arlington, VA: American Psychiatric Press, Inc.

Dorahy, M. J., Irwin, H. J., & Middleton, W. (2002). Cognitive inhibition in dissociative identity disorder (DID): Developing an understanding of working memory function in DID. *Journal of Trauma and Dissociation, 3,* 111-132.

Dorahy, M. J., Irwin, H. J., & Middleton, W. (2004). Assessing markers of working memory function in dissociative identity disorder using neutral stimuli: A comparison with clinical and general population samples. *Australian and New Zealand Journal of Psychiatry, 38,* 47-55.

Dorahy, M. J., McCusker, C. G., Loewenstein, R. J., Colbert, K., & Mulholland, C. (2006) Cognitive inhibition and interference in dissociative identity disorder: The effects of anxiety on specific executive functions. *Behaviour Research and Therapy, 44,* 749-764.

Dorahy, M. J., Middleton, W., & Irwin, H. J. (2004). Investigating cognitive inhibition in dissociative identity disorder compared to depression, posttraumatic stress disorder and schizophrenia. *Journal of Trauma and Dissociation, 5,* 93-110.

Dorahy, M. J., Middleton, W., & Irwin, H. J. (2005). The effect of emotional context on cognitive inhibition and attentional processing in dissociative identity disorder. *Behaviour Research and Therapy, 43,* 555-568.

Dorahy, M. J., & Van der Hart, O. (in press). Trauma and Dissociation: An historical perspective. In E. Vermetten, M. J. Dorahy, & D. Spiegel (Eds.), *Traumatic Dissociation: Neurobiology and Treatment.* Arlington, VA: American Psychiatric Publishing, Inc.

Ehlers, A., & Clark, D. M. (2000). A cognitive model of posttraumatic stress disorder. *Behaviour Research and Therapy, 38*, 319-345.

Elzinga, B. M., Phaf, R. H., Ardon, A. M., & Van Dyck, R. (2003). Directed forgetting between, but not within, dissociative personality states. *Journal of Abnormal Psychology, 112*, 237-243.

Elzinga, B. M., De Beurs, E., Sergeant, J. A., Van Dyck, R., & Phaf, R. H. (2000). Dissociative style and directed forgetting. *Cognitive Therapy and Research, 24*, 279-295.

Foa, E. B., & Hearst-Ikeda, D. (1996). Emotional dissociation in response to trauma: An information-processing approach. In L. K. Michelson & W. J. Ray (Eds.), *Handbook of dissociation: Theoretical, empirical and clinical perspectives* (pp. 207-224). New York: Plenum Press.

Fox, E. (1995). Negative priming from ignored distractors in visual selection: A review. *Psychonomic Bulletin and Review, 2*, 145-173.

Fox, E. (1996). Selective processing of threatening words in anxiety: The role of awareness. *Cognition and Emotion, 10*, 449-480.

Freud, S. (1926/2001). Inhibitions, symptoms and anxiety. In J. Strachey (ed.), *Standard edition of the complete psychological works of Sigmund Freud, 20* (pp. 87-175). London: Hogarth.

Freyd, J. J. (1996). *Betrayal trauma: The logic of forgetting childhood abuse.* Cambridge, MA: Harvard University Press.

Freyd, J. J., Martorello, S. R., Alvarado, J. S., Hayes, A. E., & Christman, J. C. (1998). Cognitive environments and dissociative tendencies: Performance on the standard Stroop task for high versus low dissociators. *Applied Cognitive Psychology, 12*, S91-S103.

Giesbrecht, T., Merckelbach, H., Geraerts, E., & Smeets, E. (2004). Dissociation in undergraduate students: Disruptions in executive functioning. *Journal of Nervous and Mental Disease, 192*, 567-569.

Gershuny, B.S., Cloitre, M., & Otto, M.W. (2003). Peritraumatic dissociation and PTSD severity: Do event-related fears about death and control mediate their relation? *Behaviour Research and Therapy, 41*, 157-166.

Hasher, L., & Zacks, R. T. (1988). Working memory, comprehension and aging: A review and a new view. In G. Bower (Ed.), *The psychology of learning and motivation: Advances in research and theory* (pp. 193-225). San Diego: Springer-Verlag.

Hermans, E. J., Nijenhuis, E. R. S., Van Honk, J., Hunjens, R. J. C., & Van der Hart, O. (2006). Identity state-dependent attentional bias for facial threat in dissociative identity disorder. *Psychiatry Research, 141*, 233-236.

Hilgard, E. R. (1986). *Divided consciousness: Multiple controls in human thought and action.* New York: Wiley.

Hilgard, E. R. (1994). Neodissociation theory. In S. J. Lynn & J. W. Rhue (Eds.), *Dissociation: Clinical and Theoretical Perspectives* (pp. 32-51). New York: Guilford Press.

Holmes, E. A., Brewin, C. R., & Hennessy, R. G. (2004). Trauma films, information processing, and intrusive memory development. *Journal of Experimental Psychology: General, 133*, 3-22.

Holmes, E. A., Brown, R. J., Mansell, W., Fearon, R. P., Hunter, E. C. M., Frasquilho, F., & Oakley, D. A. (2005). Are there two qualitatively distinct forms of dissociation? A review and some clinical implications. *Clinical Psychology Review, 25,* 1-23.

Huntjens, R. J. C., Postma, A., Peters, M. L., Woertman, L., & van der Hart, O. (2003). Interidentity amnesia for neutral, episodic information in dissociative identity disorder. *Journal of Abnormal Psychology, 112,* 290-297.

Irwin, H. J. (1998). Affective predictors of dissociation-II: Shame and guilt. *Journal of Clinical Psychology, 54,* 237-245.

Janet, P. (1907). *The major symptoms of hysteria.* London/New York: Macmillan. Reprint of 1920 edition: New York: Hafner, 1965.

Kennedy, F., Clarke, S., Stopa, L., Bell, L., Rouse, H., Ainsworth, C., Fearon, P., & Waller, G. (2004). Towards a cognitive model and measure of dissociation. *Journal of Behavior Therapy and Experimental Psychiatry, 35,* 25-48.

Kihlstrom, J. F. (1987). The cognitive unconscious. *Science, 237,* 1445-1452.

Kindt, M., & Van den Hout, M. (2003). Dissociation and memory fragmentation: Experimental effects on meta-memory but not on actual memory performance. *Behaviour Research and Therapy, 41,* 167-178.

Kluft, R. P. (1990). Dissociation and subsequent vulnerability: A preliminary study. *Dissociation, 3,* 167-173.

Ludwig, A. M. (1983). The psychobiological functions of dissociation. *American Journal of Clinical Hypnosis, 26,* 93-99.

Mathews, A., & MacLeod, C. (1985). Selective processing of threat cues in anxiety states. *Behaviour Research and Therapy, 23,* 563-569.

Matthews, G., & Harley, T. A. (1996). Connectionist models of emotional distress and attentional bias. *Cognition and Emotion, 10,* 561-600.

Matthews, G., & Wells, A. (1999). The cognitive science of attention and emotion. In T. Dalgleish & M. Power (Eds.), *Handbook of cognition and emotion* (pp. 171-192). Chichester: Wiley.

McNally, R. J., Kaspi, S. P., Reimann, B. C., & Zeitlin, S. B. (1990). Selective processing of threat cues in posttraumatic stress disorder. *Journal of Abnormal Psychology, 99,* 398-402.

Neill, W. T. (1977). Inhibitory and facilitatory processes of selective attention. *Journal of Experimental Psychology: Human Perception and Performance, 3,* 444-450.

Simeon, D., Knutelska, M. E., Putnam, F. W., Schmeidler, J., & Smith, L. (November, 2005). *Attention and memory in dissociative disorder, posttraumatic stress disorder, and healthy volunteers.* Paper presented at the 22nd Annual conference of the International Society for the Study of Dissociation. Toronto, Canada.

Spiegel, D. (1986). Dissociating damage. *American Journal of Clinical Hypnosis, 29,* 123-131.

Steele, K., Van der Hart, O., & Nijenhuis, E.R.S. (2005). Phase-oriented treatment of structural dissociation in complex traumatization: Overcoming trauma-related phobias. *Journal of Trauma and Dissociation, 6,* 11-53.

Stroop, J. R. (1935). Studies of interference in serial verbal reactions. *Journal of Experimental Psychology, 18,* 643-662.

Tipper, S. P., & Cranston, M. (1985). Selective attention and priming: Inhibitory and facilitatory effects of ignored primes. *Quarterly Journal of Experimental Psychology, 37A,* 591-611.

Vaillant, G.E. (1992). The historical origins of Sigmund Freud's concept of the mechanisms of defense. In G.E. Vaillant (Ed.), *Ego mechanisms of defense: A guide for clinicians and researchers* (pp. 3-28). Washington, DC: American Psychiatric Press, Inc.

Van der Hart, O., Nijenhuis, E.R.S., & Steele, K. (2006). *The haunted self: Structural dissociation and the treatment of chronic traumatization.* London: Norton.

Veltman, D. J., De Ruiter, M. B., Rombouts, S. A. R. B., Lazeron, R. H. C., Barkhof, F., Van Dyck, R., Dolan, R. J., & Phaf, R. H. (2004). Neurophysiological correlates of increased verbal working memory in high-dissociative participants: A functional MRI study. *Psychological Medicine, 35,* 175-185.

Watts, F. N., McKenna, F. P., Sharrock, R., & Trezise, L. (1986). Colour naming of phobia-related words. *British Journal of Psychology, 77,* 97-108.

Waller, G., Quinton, S., & Watson, D. (1995). Dissociation and the processing of threat-related information. *Dissociation, 8,* 84-90.

Wells, A., & Matthews, G. (1994). *Attention and emotion: A clinical perspective.* Hillsdale, NJ: Lawrence Erlbaum Associates.

Winnicott, D. W. (1945). Primitive Emotional Development. *The International Journal of Psycho-analysis, 26,* 137-143.

Williams, J. M. G., Mathews, A., MacLeod, C. (1996). The emotional Stroop task and psychopathology. *Psychological Bulletin, 120,* 3-24.

Wood, J., Mathews, A., & Dalgleish, T. (2001) Anxiety and cognitive inhibition. *Emotion, 1,* 166-181.

doi:10.1300/J229v07n04_03

A Model of Dissociation
Based on Attachment Theory and Research

Giovanni Liotti, PhD

SUMMARY. The article offers an historical review of studies on the role played by attachment processes in dissociative psychopathology. The treatise proceeds from Bowlby's first insights, through Main and her collaborators' empirical studies on attachment disorganization, to the first formulation of the hypothesis linking disorganized early attachment to pathological dissociation. Recent research supporting the hypothesis is then reviewed. It is concluded that infant attachment disorganization is in itself a dissociative process, and predisposes the individual to respond with pathological dissociation to later traumas and life stressors. Four implications of this theory are interspersed in the review and are discussed in the final section: (1) pathological dissociation should be viewed as a primarily intersubjective reality hindering the integrative processes of consciousness, rather than as an intrapsychic defense against mental pain; (2) early defenses against attachment-related dissociation are based on interpersonal controlling strategies that inhibit the attachment system; (3) dissociative symptoms emerge as a consequence of the collapse of these defensive strategies in the face of events that powerfully activate the attachment system; (4) psychotherapy of pathological dissociation should be a phase-oriented process focused primarily on achieving attachment security, and only secondarily on

Address correspondence to: Giovanni Liotti, Scuola di Psicoterapia Cognitiva, Roma, Viale Castro Pretorio, 116, 00185 Roma (Italy) (E-mail office: liotti@apc.it, E-mail home: gio.liotti@fastwebnet.it).

[Haworth co-indexing entry note]: "A Model of Dissociation Based on Attachment Theory and Research." Liotti, Giovanni. Co-published simultaneously in *Journal of Trauma & Dissociation* (The Haworth Medical Press, an imprint of The Haworth Press, Inc.) Vol. 7, No. 4, 2006, pp. 55-73; and: *Exploring Dissociation: Definitions, Development and Cognitive Correlates* (ed: Anne P. DePrince, and Lisa DeMarni Cromer) The Haworth Medical Press, an imprint of The Haworth Press, Inc., 2006, pp. 55-73. Single or multiple copies of this article are available for a fee from The Haworth Document Delivery Service [1-800-HAWORTH, 9:00 a.m. - 5:00 p.m. (EST). E-mail address: docdelivery@haworthpress.com].

Available online at http://jtd.haworthpress.com
doi:10.1300/J229v07n04_04

trauma work. Research studies on the psychotherapy process could test some predictions of this model. doi:10.1300/J229v07n04_04 *[Article copies available for a fee from The Haworth Document Delivery Service: 1-800-HAWORTH. E-mail address: <docdelivery@haworthpress.com> Website: <http://www.HaworthPress.com> © 2006 by The Haworth Press, Inc. All rights reserved.]*

KEYWORDS. Attachment disorganization, controlling strategies, defenses, dissociation, mental pain

Bowlby (1973) first hinted at the relationship between attachment processes and dissociative psychopathology when he examined the possibility that unhappy care-seeking interactions with the primary caregivers could cause the infant to develop multiple internal representations of self and attachment figures instead of unitary or cohesive and secure attachments. Bowlby (1973) referred to these internal representations as Internal Working Models (IWM). In the case of multiple IWMs Bowlby explained that one IWM becomes dominant in regulating interpersonal perceptions and emotions, while the other IWMs remain segregated (or as Pierre Janet would have said, disaggregated) from mainstream conscious experience. In stressful circumstances, the segregated IWM may surface to regulate emotions and cognitions in a way that is alien to the person's usual sense of self (Bowlby, 1973). In describing a patient characterized by symptoms that we would nowadays term dissociative (derealization and depersonalization), Bowlby (1979) explained the patient's symptoms as the outcome of attachment figures subtly inducing the child to disown personal, first-hand experiences and instead to accept a false version of important attachment experiences. Bowlby's early discussion of dissociation and attachment is the beginning of a long line of inquiry with both empirical and theoretical implications for the understanding of dissociative psychopathology. The first three sections of this paper summarize this inquiry. The fourth discusses the implications of an attachment-based model of dissociation.

THE FIRST EMPIRICAL STUDIES

In 1985, Main and collaborators published a preliminary report that provided empirical evidence that some infants constructed a multiple and disaggregated IWM of self and of a *single* (often traumatized) caregiver (Main, Kaplan & Cassidy, 1985). This research identified a new, disorganized category of infant attachment (Main & Solomon, 1990), which was added to the three organized categories: secure, insecure-avoidant, insecure-resistant (Ainsworth, Blehar, Waters & Wall, 1978).

Disorganized attachment (DA) was coded in Ainsworth's classic *Strange Situation Procedure* (SSP: Ainsworth et al., 1978) when the child demonstrated lack of orientation during attachment interactions and/or incompatible responses to episodes of separation-reunion with the caregiver, emitted either simultaneously or in quick succession. DA was characterized by simultaneous approach and avoidance of the caregiver, resulting in a lack of organization and orientation in the infant's overall attachment behavior. In comparison, secure, avoidant, and resistant patterns of attachment involved a precise behavioral and attentional strategy that was easily identifiable. DA was statistically linked to *unresolved* traumas and losses in the life of the caregivers (Main & Solomon, 1990), a finding that was replicated in a large number of controlled studies (for a review, see Lyons-Ruth & Jacobvitz, 1999; for a meta-analysis, see van IJzendoorn, 1995). Not surprisingly, the percentage of infant DA classifications rose sharply from 15% in non-clinical low-risk samples to over 70% in high risk samples (e.g., samples at risk for emotional disorders, clinical samples, and family violence samples: Lyons-Ruth & Jacobvitz, 1999; Solomon & George, 1999).

Main and Hesse (1990) hypothesized that infant DA is related to a traumatized parent's care giving attitude that is frightening to the child. Children can be frightened if the caregiver's attitude is violent or if the parent's attitude expresses fear. Caregivers communicating fear and aggression in situations otherwise devoid of danger, yield "fright without solution" in infants because "the caregiver simultaneously becomes the source and the solution of the infant's alarm" (Main & Hesse, 1990, p. 163). A fright without solution interaction, even when devoid of violence or abuse, is akin to a traumatic event. Thus, fright without solution is conceptualized here as an early *relational* trauma (Schore, 2003), typical of the intergenerational transmission of traumas.

Main (1991) argued that DA involves the early construction in the infant's mind of multiple, incoherent, *disaggregated* representations of aspects of reality (the self and a single caregiver) that are otherwise represented as singular and coherent in babies with organized attachment patterns (both secure and insecure). In response to this claim, Liotti, Intreccialagli and Cecere (1991) performed a case-control study involving retrospective evidence of losses in the life of the mothers of adult dissociative patients. They assessed mothers' experiences of having a close relative die within two years of having given birth to the patients. Retrospective evidence of loss was collected in 62% of the 46 dissociative patients compared to only 13% in the control group. Since the losses in the life of the patients' primary caregivers were arguably unresolved in the period when the patients' early attachments were shaped, these losses may have contributed to the emergence of DA in a disproportionately high percentage of dissociative patients.

CLINICAL HYPOTHESES

Liotti (1992, 1994, 1995, 1999) speculated about the qualitative aspects of consciousness in DA. Multiple, simultaneous, reciprocally incompatible and disaggregated representations of self and of a *single* caregiver that are constructed *in the same environmental-emotional context* may be matched with the well known observation that infants older than 20 weeks respond with alarm and confusion to multiple images of mother projected in an arrangement of mirrors. While younger infants are not troubled by simultaneous multiple *perceptual* images of the mother, older infants are (Bower, 1971). This finding suggests that the integrative power of attention, memory and consciousness increases gradually between 6 and 18 months (Lewis & Brooks-Gunn, 1979), during the same period in which the infants' attachment bond is constructed. The simultaneous multiple *emotional* perception of self and the caregiver in DA could exceed the integrative power of consciousness in this developmental period, just as the multiple simultaneous *visual* perception of the mother in Bower's experiment does. The disorganized infant may experience an altered consciousness, akin to the trance state that results from the multiple presentations of incompatible information in the confusion technique of hypnotic induction (Erickson, 1964). Early DA, thus, comprises two fundamental aspects of dissociation: an unusual quality of conscious experience (i.e., a trance-like state) and the simultaneous multiple representations of aspects of reality normally construed as unitary.

On the basis of these speculations, Liotti (1992) proposed that DA may be the first step in different developmental pathways, leading to: (1) satisfactory adaptation (e.g., when corrective influences on the early disorganized IWM were exerted by later secure attachment experiences and no severe trauma intervened); (2) relatively minor disturbances implying only an increased propensity toward dissociation (e.g., both absence of later traumas and of corrective relational experiences); or (3) dissociative disorders (e.g., because of later traumas confirming and amplifying the dissociative features of early DA). In later papers, Liotti (1995, 1999, 2000, 2004) proposed an attachment-based model of the dissociative disorders and of other trauma-related disorders that involve dissociation, such as Borderline Personality Disorder (BPD) and complex Post-Traumatic Stress Disorder (PTSD). Liotti (1995, 1999, 2000) suggested that the dynamic shifts among the multiple, dramatic and reciprocally disaggregated representations of the disorganized IWM could be captured, in a clinically useful way, through the metaphor of Karpman's (1968) drama triangle. In the drama triangle, the interactions between the main characters oscillate between the reciprocal prototypic roles of the powerful benevolent rescuer, the equally powerful but malevolent persecutor, and the helpless victim.

IWM in infancy relies on implicit memory (Amini, Lewis, Lannon, Louie, Baumbacher, McGuinnes & Zirker, 1996); that is, memory that does not require language or consciousness. During development, part of the formerly implicit IWM may become explicit and enter both in the consciously held meanings attributed to attachment needs and into the narratives of autobiographic memory. Once the attachment system is activated (attachment is related to an inborn evolved control system that is activated by distressing experiences throughout the life span: Bowlby, 1969/1982), the IWM guides both attachment behavior and the appraisal of attachment emotions in self and others. The literature on attachment (for reviews, see Cassidy & Shaver, 1999) provides abundant evidence that the secure IWM leads to positive appraisals of one's own attachment emotions, and expectations that one's need for help and comfort will be met by significant others as a legitimate request. An insecure organized IWM (avoidant or resistant) leads to negative appraisals of attachment emotions, and expectations that one's need for help and comfort will be met as a nuisance (avoidant attachment) or as intrusive or in an unpredictable way (resistant attachment). The disorganized IWM leads to multiple, contradictory, reciprocally disaggregated (i.e., fear without solution) appraisals and expectations.

The metaphor of the drama triangle suggests that a disorganized child construes attachment interactions as shifting representations of both the attachment figure and the self as each other's persecutor, rescuer and victim. The child represents the attachment figure negatively, as the cause of the child's ever-growing fear, and positively, as a rescuer. The caregiver, notwithstanding the frightening attitude caused by unresolved traumatic memories, is usually willing to offer comfort to the child; thus, the child may feel comfort in conjunction with the fear. The IWM of DA also conveys a negative representation of a powerful, evil self meeting a fragile or even devitalized attachment figure (persecutor self, held responsible for the emotional distress and the fear expressed by the attachment figure). Moreover, the child may represent both the self and the attachment figure as helpless victims of a mysterious, invisible source of danger. Finally, because contact with the child may have comforted the distressed caregiver, the implicit memories of DA may also convey the possibility of construing the self as the powerful rescuer of a fragile adult.

The three positions of the drama triangle correspond to the three main types of alternate ego states or personalities (alters) in the Dissociative Identity Disorder (DID): persecutor alters, protective alters that act as rescuers in the face of the patients' limitations, and child (victim) alters that preserve memories of having been the helpless victims of abuse (see Ross, 1989, for a clinical discussion of the prevalence of these three types of alters in the vast array of dissociated ego states observed in DID). In the psychotherapy process, the metaphor of the drama triangle provides a unitary explanation, related to the dynamics of a single motivational system, for the quickly shifting multiple transferences that are typical in dissociative and borderline patient's psychotherapy. That is, multiple transferences are regarded as different but interrelated manifestations of the same underlying mental state: a frightened, desperate, often unconscious longing for help (Liotti, 1995).

Other clinicians have proposed different ways of conceptualizing the influence of DA in psychotherapy with dissociative and borderline patients that are compatible with the hypothesis of the drama triangle. In more traditional psychodynamic terms, the expectation of dramatic shifts in the attitudes of the caregivers, reflecting the patients' experience of early DA, has been linked to the simultaneous operations of sadistic (persecutor role of the drama triangle) and masochistic (victim role) defenses in interpersonal relationships (Blizard, 2001). These defenses produce a relational dilemma that hinders the therapeutic process: it seems impossible to the patient to achieve both self-protection and protective closeness (Blizard, 2001). The patient may then oscillate between dependence on the therapist as rescuer, and avoidance of the therapist as persecutor ("phobia of attachment" alternating with morbid dependency: Steele, Van der Hart & Nijenhuis, 2001, pp. 83 ff).

While Liotti focused on disaggregated representations of self and caregiver typical of DA, Fonagy's research concentrated on the possibility that traumatic early attachment experiences hinder Theory of Mind, reflective self and mentalization (Fonagy, 1991, 2002). Deficits in these mental functions arising from traumatic early attachments are obstacles to the conscious integration of disaggregated (dissociated or split) mental states, and can therefore intervene in the genesis both of BPD (Fonagy, Target, Gergely, Allen & Bateman, 2003) and of dissociative disorders (Fonagy, 2002).

FURTHER EMPIRICAL STUDIES

The clinical hypotheses regarding the links between DA and dissociative psychopathology encouraged further empirical investigations. For instance, clinical hypotheses prompted Main and collaborators to make detailed analyses of the phenotypic similarities between dissociative symptoms and (1) the behavior of disorganized infants during the SSP; and (2) the features of the narratives provided by the disorganized children's caregivers during the *Adult Attachment Interview* (AAI: Hesse, 1999). These similarities suggested that dissociative processes may play a causal role both in SSP behavior and in AAI narratives (Lyons-Ruth, 2003; Main & Morgan, 1996). Hesse and van IJzendoorn (1999) provided empirical evidence supporting the causal relation between dissociative processes and unresolved mental states as assessed by the AAI.

The Minnesota Longitudinal Study (MLS)

The Minnesota Longitudinal Study (MLS) provides evidence that early DA increases vulnerability to pathological dissociation throughout personality development (Carlson, 1998; Ogawa, Sroufe, Weinfield, Carlson & Egeland, 1997). The MLS involves a non-clinical sample of 168 young adults whose attachment patterns were assessed in their second year of life. The group that had infant DA showed higher mean dissociation scores as young adults than those with other types of early attachment patterns (Ogawa et al., 1997). Within this disorganized group, those who faced later traumas during childhood and adolescence had significantly higher mean dissociation scores than those who did not face later trauma. This finding provided empirical support for Liotti's (1992) hypothesis that dissociative psychopathology is the outcome of infant DA *facilitating dissociative responses to childhood traumas*.

Carlson (1998) found that early DA was linked not only to higher ratings of dissociative behavior on the Teacher Report form of the *Child Behavior Checklist* both in elementary and high school, but also to self-reports of dissociative experiences on the *Dissociative Experience Scale* at age 19. Three adolescents in the MLS had developed dissociative disorders at the time of Carlson's inquiry; all of them had been disorganized in their infant attachment to a primary caregiver (Carlson, 1998). Lyons-Ruth (2003) emphasized findings in the MLS that suggest an equal or even more relevant role of early DA with respect to later childhood traumas, in causing dissociative psychopathology.

Retrospective Report Studies

Extending a previous retrospective study examining the etiology of dissociation (Liotti et al., 1991), a group of Italian researchers conducted two multi-center case-control studies, involving 52 dissociative patients, 66 BPD patients, and 146 psychiatric non-dissociative controls. They found support for the hypothesis that losses and severe traumatic events in the lives of the dissociative patients' mothers that took place from two years before to two years after the patients' birth were risk factors for the development of dissociative disorders (Pasquini, Liotti & The Italian Group for the Study of Dissociation, 2002) and BPD (Liotti, Pasquini & The Italian Group for the Study of Dissociation, 2000).

AAI Studies

Other studies that support the link between DA and dissociative psychopathology involve the use of the AAI in clinical samples. Two categories of AAI transcripts related to infant DA, the "unresolved" (U) and the "Cannot Classify" (CC; Hesse, 1996), are particularly interesting for the study of dissociation. The U coding reflects unresolved memories of traumas and losses emerging during the AAI. The CC category is coded when they express deeply divided states of mind concerning attachment. CC interviews portray a dismissing attitude toward attachment in the first half of the transcript, and a preoccupied state of mind concerning attachment in the second half (or vice versa), without any hint that the respondent is aware of the change in attitude during the interview. These interviews cannot be classified as "dismissing" or "preoccupied" and they obviously do not portray a secure state of mind concerning attachment. Most CC interviews are also rated high for unresolved traumas and/or losses (Hesse, 1996; Steele & Steele, 2003). Interestingly, participants whose interviews are coded CC have infants whose attachment is coded as disorganized in the SSP. U and CC codes are particularly frequent in clinical, dissociative and borderline samples however they are not rare in non-clinical, low-risk samples. This hints at the presence of sub-clinical but clearly problematic dissociative processes in the general population.

Several studies point to links between U or CC coding and dissociative symptoms. West, Adam, Spreng and Rose (2001) found that dissociative symptoms were more frequent among 69 adolescent psychotherapy patients whose AAI was coded U or CC (disorganized group) compared to a control group of 64 adolescent psychotherapy patients whose AAI coding was unrelated to DA. Barone (2003) found a significantly higher percentage of U coding in the AAI of BDP patients in a comparison to a non-clinical control group. Steele and Steele (2003) reported preliminary findings of a clinical study of dissociative patients involving the AAI that show a high percentage of CC interviews in this clinical population.

When used with patients suffering from DID, the AAI regularly elicits multiple narratives, and sometimes multiple narrating voices, in the same individual (Steele & Steele, 2003). These multiple narratives reflect distinct ego states, or personality organizations, each with a different mental state concerning attachment. Not infrequently in this clinical sample, a switch in ego state signals the narration of a horrifying history of abuse suffered at the hand of an attachment figure that is not accessible to the preceding ego state. Steele and Steele (2003) call attention to an important observation: "while psychic pain certainly accompanies the recall of the abuse per se, this pales in comparison to the much greater pain that accompanies the recall of being betrayed by trusted caregivers and siblings" (Steele & Steele, 2003, pp. 116-117). That is, the memory of an attachment figure who fails to protect the child from the abuse perpetrated by another member of the family may be more painful than the memory of the abuse per se. From an attachment theory perspective, the abused child is forced by the inborn propensity to preserve the attachment relationship and to trust the caregiver and may therefore collude with a parent's denial of the abuse perpetrated by another member of the family: this collusion implies dissociation of the traumatic memory (Bowlby, 1988, pp. 99-118; Freyd, 1997).

Besides the U and CC, a new coding system for the AAI promises to be of great interest in the study of the relations between DA and dissociation (Lyons-Ruth, Yellin, Melnick & Atwood, 2003). In the attempt to account for those instances of disorganized infant attachment that are *not* linked to caregivers' unresolved (U) mental states (a substantial minority in the first AAI-SSP studies), Lyons-Ruth and her collaborators developed a system for coding separately AAI interviews reporting multiple and non-integrated mental states both in self and in the attachment figures, but not *unresolved* memories of traumas and losses. The disaggregated mental states are alike to the drama triangle, being characterized by hostility (persecutor), helplessness (victim) and compulsively caregiving (rescuer) attitudes toward parents (Lyons-Ruth, 2003; Lyons-Ruth et al., 2003). The code for these disaggregated representations of self and the attachment figures is called "hostile–helpless" (HH). Preliminary findings of researches using the new system indicate that HH codes are linked to the vast majority (over 90%) both of infant DAs in the SSP and of borderline diagnoses in a clinical sample comparing dysthymic and BPD patients (Lyons-Ruth et al., 2003; Melnick, Lyons-Ruth, Hobson & Patrick, 2003).

Child-Caregiver Interactions Responsible for DA

In the last decade, a number of empirical studies have provided support for Main and Hesse's (1990) hypothesis that the relationship between unresolved states of mind in the caregiver and DA in the infant was mediated by frightened and frightening parental behavior. Home based observations of mother-infant interactions showed that infant disorganized behavior immediately followed mother's abrupt expressions of fear, worried absorption in internal states, or rage (Hesse, Main, Abrams & Rifkin, 2003). These studies provided some disquieting examples of disturbed parent-infant interactions in low-risk samples and illustrated how parent's attitudes can induce fright without solution and dissociative reactions in the infant *even when the parents' behavior did not constitute maltreatment* in the usual sense of the term. For instance, while seemingly trying to soothe the infant's cry, an unresolved parent approached her child from behind and slid both hands around the infant's neck. Other parents froze with a "dead" stare, unblinking in the face of the infant's cry for help. Some parents manifested a paradoxically deferential attitude toward the infant. Still others seemed to seek comfort from the infant, in a patent inversion of the attachment relationship (Hesse et al., 2003).

Childhood Sequels of Infant DA

There is evidence that, in the absence of further traumatic experiences, parents and children involved in the type of interaction that leads to infant DA tend to develop more organized and coherent strategies for daily exchanges over the ensuing two to four years. These strategies, however, do not correct the underlying disorganization. In order to understand how these strategies are developed, it is useful to keep in mind that human interpersonal relationships are regulated by different evolved inborn dispositions. At least five different behavioral/motivational systems, with an inborn evolved basis, regulate attachment (care-seeking), care-giving, social ranking, sexual mating and cooperative types of behavior (Gilbert, 1989, 2000; Liotti, 1994, 2000).

Two prospective longitudinal studies (reviewed by Lyons-Ruth & Jacobvitz, 1999, pp. 532-533) demonstrated the shift from disorganized interaction between infant and parent to a later type of child organized behavior toward the caregiver. Over 80% of school-age children who were classified as disorganized in infancy displayed either punitive-dominant or care-giving behavior toward the attachment figure. These two attitudes have both been subsumed under the heading "controlling" because through either of them the child can exert active control on the parent's attention and behavior.

Controlling strategies imply that children, in their relation with parents, "assume a role which is usually considered more appropriate for a parent with reference to a child" (Main & Cassidy, 1988, p. 418). Children who exert control over the parent through a care-giving strategy seem to have inverted the usual direction of the attachment interaction, as if they have activated the care-giving motivational system instead of the attachment system (Solomon & George, 1999). Children who control the parent through punitive-dominant strategies activate another inborn behavioral/motivational system to substitute for the normal operations of the attachment system. Namely, they activate the evolved system that regulates interactions aimed at defining the reciprocal roles of dominance and submission in the social group (identified by ethologists as the social-ranking system: Gilbert, 1989). Thus, the interaction of controlling-punitive children with their parents is regulated more often by an aggressive striving for dominance than by care-seeking (Sloman, Atkinson, Milligan & Liotti, 2002).

Controlling strategies may be interpreted as a defensive process, safeguarding the child's family relationships from disorganization at the expense of abnormally frequent inverted care-giving or competitive interactions (Liotti, 2004). The defensive activation of another motivational system in response to a disorganized IWM of attachment, however, should not necessarily be construed as a purely intra-psychic process. Rather, empirical observations suggest that caregivers' attitudes influence the child's defensive use of motivational systems substituted for the attachment system (e.g., Hesse et al., 2003). Parents who show FF behaviors toward their (disorganized) infant children also display an unusual array of submissive, care-seeking or even sexualized behaviors (Hesse et al., 2003).

The competitively aggressive, inverted care-giving or sexualized interactions between child and parent *limit* the influence of the IWM on the child's current thought, emotion and behavior by substituting for the activation of the attachment system (Liotti, 2000, 2002). These interactions, however, do not cancel the disorganized IWM from the child's mind. The disorganized IWM becomes manifest again when the child's attachment system is activated by conditions that are able to overcome the relative inhibition. For instance, 6 year old controlling children appeared well oriented and organized in their thinking, behavior, and attention until they were shown pictures from a *Separation Anxiety Test* (Hesse et al., 2003). These pictures portrayed situations that activated the child's attachment system (e.g., parents leaving a child alone). Once the system was activated, the controlling strategy collapsed, and the children revealed their underlying disorganization by providing incoherent, unrealistic, catastrophic narratives in response to the pictures. This illustrated an important process in the pathogenesis of trauma-related disorders based on a disorganized IWM. The relative inhibition of the attachment system through the defensive activation of other equally inborn motivational systems (the care-giving, the social-ranking, and/or perhaps the sexual system, as may occur in some sexually abusive families) was suspended under the influence of a powerful stressor. The coherence of thought, emotion and behavior that was secured by the defensive motivational systems disappeared. The intrinsically dissociative IWM of DA intervened (together with the emotions evoked by the stressor) in determining the dissociative response. This type of pathogenic process may explain the intriguing cases of delayed manifestation or exacerbation of dissociative disorders years after the original traumatic experience without any repetition of the original trauma. In order to bring out previously latent dissociative tendencies, any event that could either strongly activate attachment needs or invalidate controlling strategies may be sufficient (Liotti, 2004).

IMPLICATIONS OF AN ATTACHMENT BASED MODEL OF DISSOCIATION

The model of dissociative psychopathology emerging from attachment theory and research cannot solve the age-old problem, whether "the self is not a pristine unity but an entity achieved by integration of simultaneous psychological existences," or "the self is a pristine unity but uses defenses which have the effect of dysunification" (Rycroft, 1987, p.198). One cannot prove false the hypothesis that DA is the result of archaic defenses against the unbearable mental pain of fright without solution, and that these defenses yield fragmentation of a previously unitary self already present at birth. It seems, however, more plausible that DA reflects not the outcome of defenses, but an intersubjective failure of the integrative processes that normally *create* a unitary sense of self during the first year of life–a self that is absent at birth.

The prevailing contemporary theories of neonatal consciousness (e.g., Meares, 2005; Schore, 2003; Stern, 1986) suggest that in the self-organizing brain (Edelman & Tononi, 2000) of newborn infants integrative processes that *tend* to create a unitary sense of self and later on a unitary self-representation are already operant, but only at the implicit, radically intersubjective level of mental processes. During the first year of life, the self-organizing brain realizes such a tendency and yields a unitary self-representation only in securely attached infants and, to a lesser degree, in organized insecure attachments. In DA, the tendency to integrate multiple information into a unitary self-representation fails. This implies that a dissociative mind (Howell, 2005) emerges, at the beginning of life, in conjunction with operations of the attachment system, not in moments of the infant-caregiver interactions that are regulated by a motivational system different from attachment. Dissociative phenomena never arise as a function of the only other inborn interpersonal system that, alternating with the attachment system, is active since the very beginning of life: the cooperative and intersubjective system regulating parent-infant play and proto-conversations (Trevarthen, 1974).

The care-seeking-caregiving interactions between disorganized infants and their parents are heavily influenced by dissociative processes and are linked to the caregivers' unresolved traumas and losses. Caregiver's dissociation interacts in a self-perpetuating loop with the ongoing dissociative processes in the infant's mind. Dissociation, at least at the beginning of life, appears therefore to be grounded in interpersonal, dialogic processes (Lyons-Ruth, 2003) rather than in intrapsychic defenses against mental pain. This statement does not rule out the possibility that individual risk factors play a role in dissociation. It asserts, however, that individual (genetic, neurological) risk factors can yield pathological dissociation only through the mediation of dialogical processes such as those of DA. The reader interested in the interplay between interpersonal processes, individual genetics and brain functions in the genesis of DA may profit form consulting recent papers by Buchheim and George (in press), Henninghausen and Lyons-Ruth (2005), and Schore (2003).

The inborn tendency of mental operations toward unity does not disappear in disorganized infants. Before they reach school-age, the majority of children who were disorganized infants achieve a unitary type of interpersonal behavior toward their caregivers and a unitary, albeit unstable, self-representation (Lyons-Ruth & Jacobvitz, 1999, p. 532 ff). These children attempt to control the relationship with caregivers through attitudes that are typical of parents toward their babies (dominant-punitive or care-giving attitudes). The emerging controlling strategy is based on the inhibition of the attachment system through the activation of a different interpersonal motivational system (see paragraph 3.4.). Children's behavior may be interpreted as a defense against the unbearable feeling of disorientation and disorganization linked to fright without solution. Thus, the child' behavior serves as a defense *against* dissociation (which in turn should be interpreted as a primarily intersubjective process), rather than dissociation serving primarily as a defense against mental pain. Whenever mental pain activates the attachment system, the dissociative processes linked to the disorganized IWM emerge in consciousness and disrupt the integrative power of consciousness, as the consequence of a collapse or failure of the defensive controlling strategies rather than as a primary defense against mental pain. Thus, an attachment-based model of dissociation supports Janet's rather than Freud's view on the unity of the self: unity of self-representation, rather than being pristine, is achieved though integrative processes, and defenses do not play a primary role in fragmentation of the self throughout childhood. Dissociation may be *secondarily* used as a defense against mental pain in later developmental stages. Secondary, intrapsychic and defensive use of dissociation may occur when the implicit knowledge of dissociative mental states that originally were intersubjective becomes the basis for avoiding unpleasant experiences in a difficult environment, e.g., by absorbing oneself in a trance-like state.

An attachment-based model of dissociation fits with a phase-oriented, contextual psychotherapy for the dissociative disorders where trauma-work is secondary to achieving security in the therapeutic and other significant interpersonal relationships (e.g., Courtois, 1997; Gold, Elhai, Rea, Weiss, Masino, Morris & McInich, 2001; Liotti, Mollon & Miti, 2005). Therefore, future research on the process of phase-oriented psychotherapy could test some predictions of the attachment-based theory of dissociation. An example is the prediction that dissociative patients typically show, in their behavior toward the psychotherapist, multiple representations of self-with-other that shift among the poles of the drama triangle (Liotti, 1995). Another example is the prediction that particularly intense decreases of metacognitive capacity accompany moments when multiple transferences emerge (Fonagy, 1999; Liotti, 2004). Controlled studies that test these predictions are feasible: problematic mental states, such as the non-integrated representations of the drama triangle, and transient changes in metacognitive capacity can be both reliably assessed in transcripts of therapeutic sessions (Semerari, Carcione, Dimaggio, Falcone, Nicolò, Procacci & Alleva, 2003a, 2003b).

Researchers and clinicians still lack methods for reliably assessing the activation and de-activation of motivational systems (attachment, caregiving, competition, sexuality) within the therapeutic relationship. Thus, the critical prediction of the attachment-based model of dissociation–that dissociative experiences of clinical relevance are contingent upon the activation of the attachment system–cannot be empirically tested within the therapeutic relationship, for the time being, in any systematic way. However, careful analyses of the interpersonal contexts in which dissociative symptoms first appear in patients' lives could provide support for this and other attachment-based predictions. For example, the attachment-based theory of dissociation predicts that the interpersonal contexts in which dissociative symptoms first appear will be characterized by (1) losses and actual or expected separations from attachment figures; (2) creation of new bonds implying attachment; (3) lack of appropriate soothing responses to any type of stressor intervening in the patient's life, including traumatic stressors; (4) life experiences that invalidate defensive strategies based on compulsive care-giving or compulsive competition for social rank. The theory also predicts that controlling interpersonal strategies–based on *compulsive* care-giving, competition for social rank or sexual seductiveness–will be typically adopted by dissociative patients in periods of their lives when their explicit dissociative symptoms remit spontaneously. Data from empirical studies based on these predictions could lend support to the hypothesis that dissociative symptoms emerge not only as a reaction to traumatic experiences, but also through the mediation of a disorganized IWM that becomes active whenever mental pain activates the attachment motivational system.

REFERENCES

Ainsworth, M.D.S., Blehar, M., Waters, E. & Wall, S. (1978). *Patterns of attachment: A psychological study of the Strange Situation.* Hillsdale, NJ: Erlbaum.

Amini, F., Lewis, T., Lannon, R., Louie, A., Baumbacher, G., McGuinnes, T. & Zirker, E. (1996). Affect, attachment, memory: Contributions toward psychobiologic integration. *Psychiatry, 59,* 213-239.

Barone, L. (2003). Developmental protective and risk factors in borderline personality disorder: A study using the Adult Attachment Interview. *Attachment and Human Development, 5,* 64-77.

Blizard, R.A. (2001). Masochistic and sadistic ego states: Dissociative solutions to the dilemma of attachment to an abusive caregiver. *Journal of Trauma & Dissociation, 2,* 37-58.

Bower, T. (1971). The object in the world of the infant. *Scientific American, 225,* 30-38.

Bowlby, J. (1969/1982). *Attachment and loss. Vol.1: Attachment.* London: Hogarth Press.

Bowlby, J. (1973). *Attachment and loss, Vol. 2: Separation: Anxiety and anger.* London: Hogarth Press.

Bowlby, J. (1979). On knowing what you are not supposed to know and feeling what you are not supposed to feel. *Canadian Journal of Psychiatry, 24,* 403-408.

Bowlby, J. (1988). *A secure base: Clinical applications of attachment theory.* London: Routledge.

Buchheim, A. & George, C. (in press). The representational and neurobiological foundations of attachment disorganization in borderline personality disorder. In J. Solomon & C. George (Eds), *Disorganization of attachment and caregiving.* New York: The Guilford Press.

Cassidy, J. & Shaver, P. (Eds) (1999). *Handbook of attachment.* New York: Guilford Press.

Edelman, G. M. & Tononi, G. (2000). *A universe of consciousness.* New York: Basic Books.

Erickson, M. H. (1964). The confusion technique in hypnosis. *American Journal of Clinical Hypnosis, 6,* 183-207.

Fonagy, P. (1991). Thinking about thinking: Some clinical and theoretical considerations concerning the treatment of borderline patients. *International Journal of Psychoanalysis, 72,* 639-656.

Fonagy, P. (1999). The transgenerational transmission of holocaust trauma: Lessons learned from the analysis of an adolescent with obsessive-compulsive disorder. *Attachment and Human Development, 1,* 92-114.

Fonagy, P. (2002). Multiple voices versus meta-cognition: An attachment theory perspective. In V. Sinason (ed.), *Attachment, trauma and multiplicity*. London: Brunner/Routledge. pp. 71-85.

Fonagy, P., Target, M., Gergely, G., Allen, J.G. & Bateman, A.W. (2003). The developmental roots of borderline personality disorder in early attachment relationships: A theory and some evidence. *Psychoanalytic Inquiry, 23*, 412-459.

Freyd, J.J. (1997). *Betrayal trauma: The logic of forgetting child abuse*. Cambridge, MA: Harvard University Press.

George, C. & Solomon, J. (1999). Attachment and caregiving: The caregiving behavioral system. In Cassidy, J. & Shaver P.R. (Eds.), *Handbook of attachment*. New York: Guilford (pp. 649-671).

Gilbert, P. (1989). *Human nature and suffering*. London: LEA.

Gold, S.N., Elhai, J.D., Rea, B.D., Weiss, D., Masino, T., Morris, S.L. & McInich, J. (2001). Contextual treatment of dissociative identity disorder: Three case studies. *Journal of Trauma & Dissociation, 2*, 5-35.

Henninghausen, K.H. & Lyons-Ruth, K. (2005). Disorganization of behavioural and attentional strategies toward primary attachment figures: From biologic to dialogic processes. In S. Carter & L. Ahnert (Eds.), *Attachment and bonding: A new synthesis*, pp. 269-300. Cambridge, Mass.: The MIT Press.

Hesse, E. (1996). Discourse, memory and the Adult Attachment Interview: A note with emphasis on the emerging cannot classify category. *Infant Mental Health Journal, 17*, 4-11.

Hesse, E. (1999). The Adult Attachment Interview: Historical and current perspectives. In Cassidy, J. & Shaver P.R. (Eds.), *Handbook of attachment*. New York: Guilford, pp. 395-433.

Hesse, E., Main, M., Abrams, K.Y. & Rifkin, A. (2003). Unresolved states regarding loss or abuse can have "second-generation" effects: Disorganized, role-inversion and frightening ideation in the offspring of traumatized non-maltreating parents. In D.J. Siegel & M.F. Solomon (Eds.) *Healing trauma: Attachment, mind, body and brain*. New York: Norton, pp. 57-106.

Hesse, E. & van IJzendoorn, M.H. (1999). Propensities toward absorption are related to lapses in the monitoring of reasoning or discourse during the Adult Attachment Interview: A preliminary investigation. *Attachment and Human Development, 1*, 67-91.

Howell, E.F. (2005). *The Dissociative Mind*. Hillsdale, NJ: The Analytic Press.

Lewis, M. & Brooks-Gunn, J. (1979) *Social cognition and the acquisition of self*. New York, Plenum Press.

Liotti, G. (1992). Disorganized/disoriented attachment in the etiology of the dissociative disorders. *Dissociation, 5*, 196-204.

Liotti, G. (1994). *La dimensione interpersonale della coscienza [The interpersonal dimension of consciousness]*. Roma: NIS.

Liotti, G. (1995). Disorganized/disoriented attachment in the psychotherapy of the dissociative disorders. In S. Goldberg, R. Muir & J. Kerr (Eds.), *Attachment theory: Social, developmental and clinical perspectives*. Hillsdale, NJ: Analytic Press, pp. 343-363.

Liotti, G. (1999). Disorganized attachment as a model for the understanding of dissociative psychopathology. In: J. Solomon & C. George (Eds.), *Attachment Disorganization*. New York: Guilford Press, pp. 291-317.

Liotti, G. (2000). Disorganized attachment, models of borderline states, and evolutionary psychotherapy. In P. Gilbert, K. Bailey (Eds.) *Genes on the couch: Essays in evolutionary psychotherapy.* Hove: Psychology Press, pp. 232-256.

Liotti, G. (2004). Trauma, dissociation and disorganized attachment: Three strands of a single braid. *Psychotherapy: Theory, Research, Practice and Training, 41,* 472-486.

Liotti, G. & Intreccialagli, B. (2003). Disorganized attachment, motivational systems and metacognitive monitoring in the treatment of a patient with borderline syndrome. In Cortina, M. & Marrone, M. (Eds.) *Attachment theory and the psychoanalytic process.* London: Whurr, pp. 356-381.

Liotti G., Intreccialagli B. & Cecere F. (1991). Esperienza di lutto della madre e predisposizione ai disturbi dissociativi nella prole: uno studio caso-controllo [Losses in the mother's life and predisposition to the dissociative disorders in the offspring: A case-control study]. *Rivista di Psichiatria, 26,* 283-291.

Liotti, G., Mollon, P. & Miti, G. (2005). Dissociative disorders. In Gabbard, G., Beck, J. & Holmes, J. (Eds.) *Oxford textbook of psychotherapy.* Oxford: Oxford University Press, pp. 205-213.

Lyons-Ruth, K. (2003). Dissociation and the parent-infant dialogue: A longitudinal perspective from attachment research. *Journal of the American Psychoanalytic Association, 51,* 883-911.

Lyons-Ruth, K. & Jacobvitz, D. (1999). Attachment disorganization: Unresolved loss, relational violence and lapses in behavioral and attentional strategies. In J. Cassidy & P.R. Shaver (Eds.) *Handbook of attachment.* New York: Guilford Press, pp. 520-554.

Lyons-Ruth, K. Yellin, C., Melnick, S., & Atwood, G. (2003). Childhood experiences of trauma and loss have different relations to maternal unresolved and hostile-helpless states of mind on the AAI. *Attachment and Human Development, 5,* 330-352.

Main, M. (1991). Metacognitive knowledge, metacognitive monitoring, and singular (coherent) vs. multiple (incoherent) model of attachment. in C.M.Parkes, J. Stevenson-Hinde, & P. Marris (Eds.), *Attachment across the life cycle.* Routledge, London, pp. 127-159.

Main, M. & Cassidy, J. (1988). Categories of response to reunion with the parent at age six: Predicted from infant attachment classification and stable over a one-month period. *Developmental Psychology, 24,* 415-426.

Main, M. & Hesse, E. (1990). Parents' unresolved traumatic experiences are related to infant disorganized attachment status: Is frightened and/or frightening parental behavior the linking mechanism? In M.T. Greenberg, D. Cicchetti & E.M. Cummings (Eds.), *Attachment in the preschool years.* Chicago: Chicago University Press, pp. 161-182.

Main, M. & Hesse, E.(2000). The organized categories of infant, child, and adult attachment: Flexible vs. inflexible attention under attachment-related stress. *Journal of the American Psychoanalytic Association, 48,* 1055-1095.

Main, M. & Morgan, H. (1996). Disorganization and disorientation in infant Strange Situation behavior: Phenotypic resemblance to dissociative states? In L. Michelson & W. Ray (Eds.), *Handbook of Dissociation.* New York: Plenum Press, pp.107-137.

Main, M. & Solomon, J. (1990). Procedures for identifying infants as disorganized/disoriented during the Ainsworth Strange Situation. In M.T. Greenberg, D. Cicchetti & E.M. Cummings (Eds.), *Attachment in the preschool years.* Chicago: Chicago University Press, pp. 121-160.

Meares, R. (2005). *The metaphor of play, 3rd edition.* London: Routledge.

Melnick, S. Lyons-Ruth, K. Hobson, P. & Patrick, M. (2003). *Discriminating borderline states of mind regarding attachment: Operationalizing the concepts of affective splitting and hostile-helpless states of mind on the Adult Attachment Interview.* Biennial Meeting of the Society for Research in Child Development, Tampa, FL, April, 2003.

Ogawa, J. R., Sroufe, L.A., Weinfield, N.S., Carlson, E.A. & Egeland, B. (1997). Development and the fragmented self: Longitudinal study of dissociative symptomatology in a nonclinical sample. *Development and Psychopathology, 9,* 855-879.

Pasquini, P., Liotti, G.. & The Italian Group for the Study of Dissociation (2002). Risk factors in the early family life of patients suffering from dissociative disorders. *Acta Psychiatrica Scandinavica, 105,* 110-116.

Ross, C.A. (1989). *Multiple Personality Disorder.* New York: Wiley.

Rycroft, C. (1987). Dissociation of the personality, in R. Gregory (ed.) *The Oxford companion to the mind.* Oxford: Oxford University Press, pp. 197-198.

Schore, A.N. (2003). *Affect dysregulation and disorders of the self.* Norton: New York.

Semerari, A., Carcione, A., Dimaggio, G., Falcone, M., Nicolò, G., Procacci, M. & Alleva, G. (2003a). The evaluation of metacognitive functioning in psychotherapy: The Metacognition Assessment Scale and its applications. *Clinical Psychology and Psychotherapy, 10,* 238-261.

Semerari, A., Carcione, A., Dimaggio, G., Falcone, M., Nicolò, G., Procacci, M., Alleva, G. & Mergenthaler, E. (2003b). Assessing problematic states inside patient's narratives: The grid of problematic conditions. *Psychotherapy Research, 13,* 337-353.

Sloman, L. Atkinson, L., Milligan, K. & Liotti, G. (2002). Attachment, social rank, and affect regulation: Speculations on an ethological approach to family interaction. *Family Process, 41,* 479-493.

Solomon, J. & George, C. (1999). The place of disorganization in attachment theory. In Solomon, J. & George, C. (Eds.) *Attachment disorganization.* New York: Guilford Press, pp. 3-32.

Stern, D. (1985). *The interpersonal world of the infant.* New York: Basic Books.

Steele, H. & Steele, M. (2003). Clinical uses of the Adult Attachment Interview. In Cortina, M. & Marrone, M. (Eds.) *Attachment theory and the psychoanalytic process.* London: Whurr, pp. 107-126.

Steele, K., Van der Hart, O. & Nijenhuis, E.R. (2001). Dependency in the treatment of complex posttraumatic stress disorder and dissociative disorders. *Journal of Trauma & Dissociation, 2,* 79-115.

Trevarthen, C. (1974). Conversations with a two-month-old. *New Scientist, 62,* 230-235.

van IJzendorn, M. (1995). Adult attachment representations, parental responsiveness and infant attachment: A meta-analysis of the predictive validity of the Adult Attachment Interview. *Psychological Bulletin, 117,* 387-403.

West, M., Adam, K., Spreng, S. & Rose, S. (2001). Attachment disorganization and dissociative symptoms in clinically treated adolescents. *Canadian Journal of Psychiatry, 46,* 627-631.

doi:10.1300/J229v07n04_04

Development of Dissociation: Examining the Relationship Between Parenting, Maternal Trauma and Child Dissociation

Ann Chu, MA
Anne P. DePrince, PhD

SUMMARY. While many studies have demonstrated relationships between trauma and dissociation, relatively little is known about other factors that may increase children's risk for developing dissociative symptoms. Drawing on betrayal trauma theory and Discrete Behavioral States frameworks, the current study examined the contributions of maternal factors (including mothers' dissociation, betrayal trauma experiences, and inconsistent parenting) to children's dissociation. Seventy-two mother-child dyads completed self-report questionnaires. Maternal dissociation was found to relate positively to maternal betrayal trauma his-

Ann Chu and Anne P. DePrince are affiliated with the Department of Psychology, University of Denver.

Address correspondence to: Ann Chu, Department of Psychology, University of Denver, 2155 South Race Street, Denver, CO 80208 (E-mail: achu@du.edu).

The authors offer thanks to Daniel McIntosh, Stephen Shirk, and two anonymous reviewers for comments on an earlier draft. The authors also thank Jackie Rea, Meg Saylor, and Denver social service agencies for project assistance.

This project was funded, in part, through a University of Denver Graduate Affairs Committee Research Grant (A.C.) and start-up funds (A.P.D.).

[Haworth co-indexing entry note]: "Development of Dissociation: Examining the Relationship Between Parenting, Maternal Trauma and Child Dissociation." Chu, Ann, and Anne P. DePrince. Co-published simultaneously in *Journal of Trauma & Dissociation* (The Haworth Medical Press, an imprint of The Haworth Press, Inc.) Vol. 7, No. 4, 2006, pp. 75-89; and: *Exploring Dissociation: Definitions, Development and Cognitive Correlates* (ed: Anne P. DePrince, and Lisa DeMarni Cromer) The Haworth Medical Press, an imprint of The Haworth Press, Inc., 2006, pp. 75-89. Single or multiple copies of this article are available for a fee from The Haworth Document Delivery Service [1-800-HAWORTH, 9:00 a.m. - 5:00 p.m. (EST). E-mail address: docdelivery@haworthpress.com].

tory. Additionally, both mothers' and children's betrayal trauma history were found to significantly predict children's dissociation. Implications for the intergenerational transmission of betrayal trauma and dissociation are discussed. doi:10.1300/J229v07n04_05 *[Article copies available for a fee from The Haworth Document Delivery Service: 1-800-HAWORTH. E-mail address: <docdelivery@haworthpress.com> Website: <http://www.HaworthPress. com> © 2006 by The Haworth Press, Inc. All rights reserved.]*

KEYWORDS. Dissociation, children, betrayal trauma theory, discrete behavioral states theory

Dissociation has been associated with inescapable and chronic traumas, as well as disruptions in development, including: witnessing sexual or physical abuse of family members, family disruption (removal of child from home, lack of biological mother, presence of step-father), poor parent-child interactions (avoidant and disorganized attachment, inconsistent discipline), and sexual abuse history (for reviews, see Ogawa, Sroufe, Weinfield, Carlson, & Egeland, 1997; Putnam, 1997; Silberg, 2000). Given these associations and the profound impact dissociation can have on children's development (see Putnam, 1997), researchers have begun to examine the development of dissociation in children. The current paper draws on two theories to provide a framework for testing associations between maternal factors and child dissociation: betrayal trauma theory (Freyd, 1996) and the Discrete Behavioral States model (Putnam, 1997).

Betrayal trauma theory proposes that violence perpetrated by someone on whom the victim is dependant will be associated with memory disruption, dissociation, and other cognitive dysfunctions in order to help the victim maintain the necessary, albeit abusive, attachment (see Freyd, 1996). Thus, the theory implicates dissociation as a potential mechanism in blocking trauma-related information in the case of betrayal traumas (i.e., events perpetrated by someone on whom the victim is dependent). Several studies have demonstrated that physical and sexual abuse by family members are significantly related to increased dissociation symptoms, while non-family abuse is not (Chu & Dill, 1990; Plattner, Silvermann, & Redlich, 2003). Similarly, DePrince (2005) found that reporting a betrayal trauma prior to the age of 18 was associated with pathological levels of dissociation in young adults.

The Discrete Behavioral States (DBS) model (Putnam, 1997) proposes that pathological dissociation arises from children's failure to learn to integrate states. In typical development, parents are instrumental in teaching very young children to move fluidly between states (e.g., from a distressed to a neutral state). In atypical development (such as that characterized by exposure to maltreatment or family violence), parenting factors likely mediate children's risk of developing dissociative symptoms. For example, Deblinger, Steer, and Lippmann (1999) found that children's perceptions of their mothers' parenting practices were related to children's post-trauma symptoms generally. Mann and Sanders (1994) found that dissociation was associated with parental rejection and inconsistency in applying discipline in a sample of forty boys. Ogawa et al. (1997) observed in a longitudinal study that children with disorganized or avoidant attachment styles in relating to their mothers were at higher risk for developing dissociation in adolescence. Thus, factors that affect parents' ability to help children learn to modulate states (such as parenting consistency or parent's own dissociation) may increase children's risk of developing dissociative symptoms.

MATERNAL TRAUMA HISTORY, DISSOCIATION, AND PARENTING

Earlier work suggested that women exposed to child or spousal abuse tended to engage in harsh and aggressive parenting (Jaffe, Wolfe, & Wilson, 1990). However, recent research suggests that women with abusive spouses show more behavioral inconsistency in their parenting practices compared to women without abusive spouses, rather than differences in the use of directed physical aggression or maternal authority and control (Holden & Ritchie, 1991; Holden et al., 1998; Levendosky & Graham-Bermann, 2000; Rossman & Rea, 2005). This more recent work suggests that mothers exposed to abuse may be less consistently engaged. Based on the domestic violence literature and the betrayal trauma theory framework, we expect that extent of mothers' betrayal trauma experiences would be associated with inconsistent parenting.

While much interest has focused on the parenting practices of mothers who have experienced abuse, there have been few investigations of other trauma-related factors that may have an impact on parenting, including dissociation. In one study of mothers with Multiple Personality Disorder (MPD), only 38.7% of 75 mothers qualified as competent or exceptional parents, while 45.3% were judged to be compromised or impaired, and 16.0% were abusive toward their children (Kluft, 1987). Egeland and Susman-Stillman (1996) reported that mothers abused as children who abused their own children had higher levels of dissociative symptoms than mothers abused as children who did not abuse their own children. Maternal dissociation has also been related to inconsistency in applying discipline (Collin-Vezina, Cyr, & Pauze, 2005). The disruption of typically integrated information processing in dissociation raises the possibility that highly dissociative mothers may parent their children inconsistently.

To date, inconsistent parenting has been conceptualized as lack of follow-through and inconsistency in applying discipline. However, if a parent consistently lacks follow-through and structure in their discipline, a child may reasonably predict such behaviors. On the other hand, if a parent displays behaviors that oscillate between different parenting styles, the child may have a harder time interpreting parental expectations and affective tone. In fact, results from a study conducted by Rossman and Rea (2005) suggest that inconsistencies in applying a dominant parenting style relate to higher levels of trauma symptoms in children after witnessing family violence. Thus, in this study we conceptualize inconsistent parenting as alternating between Authoritarian, Authoritative, and Permissive parenting.

CURRENT STUDY

Dissociation has been associated with chronic and inescapable trauma exposure; however, because not all trauma-exposed children experience dissociation symptoms, additional factors must also contribute to the development of dissociation. Drawing on the DBS model, we propose that maternal factors, such as mother's own dissociation and parenting inconsistency, may negatively affect children's ability to learn to modulate states, thus increasing dissociation risk. Thus, the current study examined links between maternal experiences of betrayal trauma, maternal dissociation, and inconsistent parenting practices in the prediction of child dissociation. We hypothesized that: (1) Consistent with betrayal trauma theory, extent of maternal betrayal trauma history would positively relate to maternal dissociation; (2) Mothers' dissociation would relate to differences in inconsistent parenting practices as reflected by self- and child-report on parenting questionnaires; (3) Extent of maternal betrayal trauma history would be associated with differences in inconsistent parenting; and (4) Mothers' dissociation, betrayal trauma history, and inconsistent parenting would predict children's dissociation.

METHOD

Participants

Female guardians with children (aged 7-11 years) were recruited for participation in a larger project on Parenting and Stress ($N = 72$) through flyers posted at local Denver community agencies, community centers and through the University of Denver Developmental Subject Pool. The majority of women were biological mothers to the child participant, though the sample also included adoptive mothers and one grandmother; we will refer to female guardians as mothers for the remainder of the manuscript. Five mothers did not respond regarding the child's race/ethnicity; the remaining children were reported to be of the following racial/ethnic backgrounds: 40.0% White, 18.5% Black, 18.5% Hispanic/Latino, 3.1% American Indian/Alaskan Native, 20.0% other race or bi/multiracial. One mother did not respond regarding her race; the remaining women reported the following racial/ethnic backgrounds: 44.9% White, 15.9% Black, 20.3% Hispanic/Latino, 2.9% American Indian/ Alaskan Native, 15.9% other race or bi/multiracial. See Table 1 for other relevant demographic information.

Procedure

Following informed consent procedures, mothers were asked to complete a demographics information sheet and several questionnaires to assess their trauma history, dissociation level, and parenting practices, as well as their children's dissociation level and trauma history. Children completed a questionnaire about their mothers' parenting practices. The experimenter read out loud all items on the questionnaire to the children and recorded their verbal responses on paper to ensure that reading level did not affect children's responses.

Measures

Measures of Parenting Practices. Parenting was assessed using both parent- and child-report version of the Parenting Practices Question-

TABLE 1. Demographic Information of Sample and Descriptive Statistics of Mother and Child Dissociation, Mother and Child Betrayal Trauma, and Mother Parenting Practices.

Variable	Mean (SD)	Range	Percentage
Child Age	8.73 (1.38)	7-11	
Mother Age	37.21 (7.10)	25-61	
Number of Children in Family	2.17 (0.85)	1-4	
Female Children in Sample			64.3%
Mothers Married or Living w/ Partner			46.5%
Maternal Education Level:	Some high school or GED		32.9%
	College (some or graduated)		54.3%
	Post-College		12.9%
Family Income Level	< $30,000		61.4%
	$30,000-$50,000		17.1%
	> $50,000		21.4%
Mother Dissociation	10.98 (9.94)	0.00-53.93	
Child Dissociation	5.56 (4.57)	0-24	
Mother Betrayal Trauma Sum	1.14 (1.37)	0-4	
Mother Parenting Practices (mother report/child report)			
Authoritative	4.13 (.49)/3.88 (.58)	2.74-4.96/2.37-4.81	
Authoritarian	1.90 (.41)/2.43 (.67)	1.20-3.00/1.27-3.87	
Permissive	2.05 (.47)/2.07 (.45)	1.13-3.73/1.29-3.27	

naire (PPQ; Robinson et al., 1995), a 62 item measure devised to assess Baumrind's (1967) typology of parenting styles. Factor analysis has shown the measure to be consistent with Baumrind's Authoritative, Authoritarian, and Permissive parenting typologies. Mothers were asked to indicate on a frequency scale from 1 to 5 how often they exhibited each behavior during the past year; responses from each parenting factor were then averaged to produce separate factor scores. Children indicated on a similar 5-point scale the frequency of their mothers' parenting behaviors during the past year on the PPQ-Child Version (PPQ-C). Given that both mothers and children provide unique perspectives on mother-child interactions, both reports of parenting practices were included in the analyses. Mothers may be more astute than children in reporting parenting practices; yet adults may be more sensitive to pressures of social desirability so that children may be more accurate reporters.

Using a procedure adapted from Rossman and Rea (2005), mothers were placed into parenting inconsistency groups (*highly inconsistent*, *moderately inconsistent,* and *consistent*) based on PPQ factor scores. First, high, medium, and low endorsements of each parenting factor were calculated. For mother-response, high endorsements of a parenting factor were defined as scores that fell 1/3 standard deviation above the normed mean score of that parenting factor (norms drawn from Robinson et al., 1995); medium endorsements were scores that fell within 1/3 standard deviation from the normed mean score; and low endorsements were scores that fell 1/3 standard deviation below the normed mean score. Then, mothers were assigned to the following inconsistency groups. Mothers were rated as *highly inconsistent* if they had (1) scores on at least two subscales falling in the high endorsement range or (2) medium endorsements on two subscales plus a low or medium endorsement on the remaining subscale. Mothers who had high endorsements on two of the parenting styles exhibit more than one predominant type of parenting practices. Mothers who had a medium endorsement on two or more of the subscales do not have one particular style of behaviors that they employ more dominantly than the others. Mothers were assigned to the *moderately inconsistent* group if they had either (1) one each of high, medium, and low endorsement on the three subscales or (2) high endorsement on one subscale plus medium endorsements on remaining subscales. These mothers are moderately inconsistent in their parenting because although they dominantly employ behaviors within one style most of the time, they still rely on some parenting behaviors from other parenting styles. Finally, the remaining group of mothers who were rated as consistent had low endorsements on two subscales plus moderate/high endorsement on the remaining subscale. These mothers consistently use behaviors from one style without relying on behaviors from other styles. The same procedure was used to code parenting inconsistency based on child-report data, but sample means were used instead of normed means because child norms are not available.

Measures of Dissociation. Maternal dissociation was assessed using the Dissociative Experiences Scale (DES; Bernstein & Putnam, 1986), a widely-used 28 item self-report measure. The DES has been shown to have good validity and reliability and is scored by taking an average across items. Child dissociation was assessed using the Child Dissociative Checklist (CDC; Putnam, 1993), 20-item observer-report. Participants report how much each item applies to their child on a 3-point scale. A sum of all items is calculated. The CDC has been demonstrated to have high reliability and validity (Putnam, 1993).

Measures of Trauma History. Maternal trauma history was assessed using the Trauma History Questionnaire (THQ; Green, 1996) which includes 24 behaviorally-defined items in three areas: crime-related events, general disaster and trauma, and unwanted physical and sexual experiences. Mothers indicated whether each item happened to them, and if so, the number of times and approximate age(s) of occurrence. Based on the reported relationship to the perpetrators, the total number of events that involved the betrayal of an interpersonal relationship was tallied. A dichotomous variable was also computed to indicate whether mothers experienced any betrayal trauma (yes/no). Child trauma was assessed by mother report on the UCLA-PTSD Index (Pynoos et al., 1998). Mothers indicated whether children had been exposed to 12 behaviorally-defined traumatic events; they could also write in events that were not covered by the 12 items. Children's betrayal trauma history (present/absent) was coded as present if mothers reported that the child was exposed to at least one of three abuse items or wrote in a qualifying event in response to the 'anything else' item. The three abuse items included: being hit, punched or kicked very hard at home; seeing a family member being hit, punched or kicked very hard at home; having an adult or someone much older touch your child's private sexual body parts when your child did not want them to.

RESULTS

Seventy-two mother-child dyads were tested; two mothers did not complete questionnaire packets, resulting in a final sample of 70 mother-child dyads. Differences in degrees of freedom reflect missing data on some questionnaires. See Table 1 for means (*SD*) for study variables. One outlying score on the CDC was replaced with the value of 2.5 *SD* above the mean.

PPQ scores for both mother and child reports were tallied and coded as described in the Materials section. Mother and child reports were not significantly correlated ($r = .16, p > .05$). Per mother report, mothers fell into the following groups: 20 highly inconsistent, 30 moderately inconsistent, and 20 consistent. Per child report, mothers fell into the following groups: 33 highly inconsistent, 12 moderately inconsistent, and 20 consistent.

Maternal trauma was computed based on the THQ responses. Mothers in this sample reported exposure to the following event types: 2 no trauma; 18 only non-interpersonal trauma events (i.e., accidents and natural disasters); 4 interpersonal trauma events where the relationship with the perpetrator was one of non-dependency (i.e., strangers or neighbors); 5 interpersonal trauma events where the perpetrator was one of low dependency (i.e., uncles, cousins, or grandparents); 35 interpersonal trauma events where the relationship of the perpetrator was likely to be one of high dependency (i.e., a parent or significant other). The total number of maternal betrayal trauma events (i.e., interpersonal violence in which the relationship to the perpetrator appeared to be one of high dependency) for each mother was summed; see Table 1. Mothers reported the following trauma exposure in children: 44 no betrayal trauma events and 26 at least one betrayal trauma event (9 children were reported to have more than one betrayal trauma event). For 3 out of the 26 children, mothers reported sexual abuse without specifying perpetrator relationship; in all other cases information on the UCLA-PTSD index indicated trauma as occurring within the family context.

Associations between mothers' dissociation levels, betrayal trauma history, and inconsistent parenting practices were examined. Mothers' level of dissociation was positively related to the number of betrayal trauma experiences mothers have experienced ($r = 0.34$, $p < .01$). In addition, mothers with betrayal trauma histories reported higher levels of dissociative symptoms on the DES than mothers without betrayal trauma histories ($t(61) = -2.34$, $p < .05$). Mothers with interpersonal trauma histories (regardless of betrayal in the perpetrator relationship) did not differ on dissociation from mothers without interpersonal trauma histories ($t(68) = 0.92$, $p > .05$). Neither mothers' dissociation nor mothers' betrayal trauma experiences were associated with inconsistent parenting; however, mothers' DES scores were positively related to the PPQ Permissive parenting factor score by mother report ($r = 0.42$, $p < 0.01$).

Mothers' number of betrayal trauma experiences was positively related to children's dissociation scores ($r = 0.38$, $p < .01$). Children exposed to betrayal trauma events also had higher dissociation scores on the CDC than children without betrayal trauma ($t(62) = -2.50$, $p < .05$). Children with betrayal trauma experiences had mothers who experienced more betrayal trauma events on the THQ than children without any betrayal trauma ($t(62) = -2.60$, $p < .05$).

A sequential regression was performed to determine whether mothers' dissociation, betrayal trauma history, and inconsistent parenting improved the prediction of children's dissociation levels beyond that predicted by children's trauma history. Given that mothers and children both provide unique perspectives to parenting interactions, 2 models were run separately with Model 1 based on mother-report of inconsistent parenting and Model 2 based on child-report of inconsistent parenting. Point of entry of variables remained the same for both models. Table 2 displays the unstandardized regression coefficients (B) with the standard error and the standardized regression coefficients (β) for the 2 models. In Model 1, when only child betrayal trauma had been entered, $R^2 = .07$, $F(1, 57) = 4.34$, $p < .05$. After step 2, with mother's dissociation, betrayal trauma, and inconsistent parenting (mother-report) added to the prediction of children's dissociation, $R^2 = 0.19$, $F(4, 54) = 3.10$, $p < .05$. Addition of maternal variables to the equation did not significantly improve R^2, $p = .06$. This model indicated that child betrayal trauma significantly predicted child dissociation by itself; adding maternal factors did not improve prediction of child dissociation significantly. When all predictor variables were controlled for, mothers' betrayal trauma was the only predictor variable that provided a significantly unique contribution to the prediction of child dissociation. In Model 2, when only child betrayal trauma had been entered, $R^2 = .12$, $F(1, 52) = 7.14$, $p < .01$. After step 2, with mothers' dissociation, betrayal trauma, and inconsistent parenting (child-report) added to the prediction of children's dissociation, $R^2 = .24$, $F(4, 49) = 3.95$, $p < .01$. Adding maternal variables to the equation did not significantly improve R^2, $p = .06$. This model indicated that child betrayal trauma significantly predicted child dissociation by itself; adding maternal factors did not improve the prediction significantly. When all predictor variables were included, child betrayal trauma showed only a trend in predicting child dissociation; instead, mothers' betrayal trauma provided a significantly unique contribution to this prediction.

DISCUSSION

The current study demonstrates relationships between mother and child dissociation and trauma exposure. Importantly, both mothers' and children's betrayal trauma were positively associated with children's dissociation. Regression analyses revealed that children's betrayal trauma predicted child dissociation when it was the only predictor variable in each equation. This pattern supports the association often found between dissociation and trauma experiences (e.g., Putnam, 1997). Additional maternal factors including dissociation, betrayal trauma, and inconsistent parenting did not add significantly to the prediction of chil-

TABLE 2. Summary of Sequential Regression Analysis for Variables Predicting Children's Dissociation Levels (N = 65).

Variable	B	SE B	β
Model 1			
Step 1			
Child Betrayal Trauma History	2.48	1.19	0.27*
Step 2			
Child Betrayal Trauma History	1.59	1.21	0.17
Inconsistent Parenting-Mother Report	0.74	0.79	0.12
Mother Dissociation	−0.06	0.06	−0.12
Mother Betrayal Trauma History	1.19	0.45	0.36*
Model 2			
Step 1			
Child Betrayal Trauma History	3.25	1.22	0.35**
Step 2			
Child Betrayal Trauma History	2.32	1.22	0.25+
Inconsistent Parenting-Child Report	−0.21	0.67	−0.04
Mother Dissociation	−0.02	0.07	−0.04
Mother Betrayal Trauma History	1.23	0.44	0.38**

Note. R^2 = .07 for Model 1 Step 1 ($p < .05$); R^2 = .10 for Model 1 Step 2 ($p = .09$). R^2 = .12 for Model 2 Step 1 ($p = .01$); R^2 = .12 for Model 2 Step 2 ($p = .06$). $+p = .06$, $*p < .05$, $**p < .01$.

dren's dissociation. When examining all predictor variables, only mothers' betrayal trauma contributed uniquely to the prediction of children's dissociation in both models. When the inconsistent parenting ratings based on children's report was used in Model 2, there was a trend such that children's betrayal trauma history contributed uniquely to prediction of children's dissociation. The child inconsistent parenting ratings may have had less noise than mother reports, allowing the trend to emerge in Model 2; this points to the importance of examining both mother and child reports. Taken together, both regression models suggest that while children's betrayal trauma plays an important role in predicting children's dissociation, other factors such as mothers' betrayal trauma history may also be important to consider.

The results showed an intergenerational relationship between mothers' and children's betrayal trauma histories. Children who experienced betrayal trauma had mothers who experienced higher numbers of betrayal trauma than children without betrayal trauma. It may be that mothers who have experienced betrayal traumas are, in turn, dealing with dissociative symptoms, making them less able to monitor their children and provide a safe environment.

Contrary to predictions, however, mothers' betrayal trauma history and dissociation level were not related to mothers' inconsistent parenting practices by either mother- or child-report. Inconsistent parenting did not contribute significantly to the prediction of child dissociation. Maternal dissociation was positively correlated with the Permissive parenting style (which includes inconsistent discipline in lack of follow-through) per mother report. These associations are similar to previous reported relationships between both mothers' and fathers' dissociation and inconsistent discipline (Mann & Sanders, 1994) but did not reflect the inconsistency of having different parenting styles as conceptualized in this study.

One potential mechanism for the transmission of betrayal trauma and dissociation may be alterations in information processing that could affect parenting behaviors. DePrince and Freyd (e.g., 2004) have found associations between dissociation, attention, and memory on various laboratory tasks. Additionally, DePrince (2005) found that betrayal trauma was associated with revictimization, which in turn was associated with problems detecting violations of safety and social rules. Failure to accurately process safety/social rules may leave individuals at higher risk of revictimization. With altered information processing, mothers with betrayal trauma histories or dissociative symptoms may have a harder time monitoring and creating a safe environment for their children. Thus, these children may be more likely to experience their own betrayal trauma, increasing their risk for developing dissociation. The current study did not specifically examine information processing mechanisms, pointing to the need for future research in this area.

Limitations and Future Research

We examined the relationships between child and maternal betrayal trauma history and child dissociation; however, our data did not include information on the duration, onset, and frequency of trauma in children. From a developmental psychopathology framework, the age and developmental stage when child abuse occurs should affect the posttraumatic outcomes, including the development of dissociation (Egeland & Susman-Stillman, 1996). The cross-sectional nature of the current study did not allow us to examine "sleeper effects" that might influence later development of dissociation (Finkelhor & Browne, 1985; Trickett et al., 2001).

This study relied on self-reports to assess trauma history, dissociation levels, and parenting behaviors. Although self-reports provide valuable information about the participants, they can be less reliable than direct observation or interviewing due to potential response biases or inaccurate recall of information. Child dissociation, in particular, may be difficult to assess reliably via parent report because the internal experience of dissociative symptoms may not manifest as overt behaviors in children such that mothers can observe the presence or extent of their children's dissociation (e.g., Malinosky-Rummell & Hoier, 1991). Thus, the parent-report methodology used in the current study may have limited the range of scores that were obtained for child dissociative symptoms. Mothers reported relatively low levels of dissociation for themselves and their children. In addition, most mothers endorsed items consistent with the Authoritative style of parenting. While such reporting may accurately reflect the sample tested, mothers may also have been sensitive to social desirability pressures, thus biasing their responses in a positive light. Finally, recruitment of solely mother-child dyads with the exclusion of father-child dyads prevented a complete assessment of the child's family environment.

CONCLUSION

Childhood abuse is associated with increased risk for a range of negative health outcomes, including dissociation (for a review, see Kendall-Tackett, 2002; Putnam, 1997). Thus, investigations that offer insight into the developmental impact of child maltreatment on posttraumatic symptoms, such as dissociation, remain critically important. The current study provides initial evidence that maternal betrayal trauma history may be one path through which child maltreatment and child dissociation may be transmitted intergenerationally. Mothers faced with betrayal trauma experiences and related consequences may have difficulty providing a consistent and safe environment for their children, leaving children at risk for experiencing abuse and dissociation. Thus, future research examining both parental factors (such as betrayal trauma history) and parenting practices promises to provide important insights for improving intervention and prevention programs to decrease children's risk of developing dissociation.

REFERENCES

Baumrind, D. (1967). Childcare practices anteceding three patterns of preschool behavior. *Genetic Psychology Monograph, 75*, 43-88.

Bernstein, E.M. & Putnam, F.W. (1986). Development, reliability, and validity of a dissociation scale. *Journal of Nervous and Mental Disease, 174*, 727-735.

Chu, J.A. & Dill, D.L. (1990). Dissociative symptoms in relation to childhood physical and sexual abuse. *American Journal of Psychiatry, 147*, 887-892.

Collin-Vezina, D., Cyr, M., & Pauze, R. (2005). The role of depression and dissociation in the link between childhood sexual abuse and later parental practices. *Journal of Trauma and Dissociation, 6*, 71-97.

Deblinger, E., Steer, R., & Lippmann, J. (1999). Maternal factors associated with sexually abused children's psychosocial adjustment. *Child Maltreatment: Journal of the American Professional Society on the Abuse of Children, 4*, 13-20.

DePrince, A.P. & Freyd, J. (2004). Forgetting trauma stimuli. *Psychological Science, 15*, 488-492.

DePrince, A.P. (2005). Social cognition and revictimization risk. *Journal of Trauma and Dissociation, 6*, 125-141.

Egeland, B. & Susman-Stillman, A. (1996). Dissociation as a mediator of child abuse across generations. *Child Abuse and Neglect, 20*, 1123-1132.

Finkelhor, D. & Browne, A. (1985). The traumatic impact of child sexual abuse: A conceptualization. *American Journal of Orthopsychiatry, 55*, 530-541.

Freyd, J. (1996). *Betrayal trauma: The logic of forgetting childhood abuse.* Cambridge, Massachusetts: Harvard University Press.

Green, B.L. (1996). Psychometric review of Trauma History Questionnaire (Self-report). In B.H. Stamm & E.M. Varra (Eds.), *Measurement of stress, trauma and adaptation.* Lutherville, MD: Sidran.

Holden, G.W., & Ritchie, K.L. (1991). Linking extreme marital discord, child rearing, and child behavior problems: Evidence from battered women. *Child Development, 62*, 311-327.

Holden, G.W., Stein, J.D., Ritchie, K.L., Harris, S.D., & Jouriles, E.N. (1998). Parenting behaviors and beliefs of battered women. In G.W. Holden, R. Geffner, & E.N. Jouriles (Eds.), *Children exposed to marital violence: Theory, research, and applied issues* (pp. 289-333). Washington, DC: American Psychological Association.

Jaffe, P.G., Wolfe, D.A., & Wilson, S.K. (1990). *Children of battered women.* Newbury Park, CA: Sage.

Kendall-Tackett, K. (2002). The health effects of childhood abuse: Four pathways by which abuse can influence health. *Child Abuse & Neglect, 26*, 715-729.

Kluft, R. (1987). The parental fitness of mothers with multiple personality disorder: A preliminary study. *Child Abuse and Neglect, 11*, 273-280.

Levendosky, A.A. & Graham-Bermann, S.A. (2000). Behavioral observations of parenting in battered women. *Journal of Family Psychology, 14*, 80-94.

Malinosky-Rummell, R.R. & Hoier, T.S. (1991). Validating measures of dissociation in sexually abused and nonabused children. *Behavioral Assessment, 13*, 341-357.

Mann, B.J. & Sanders, S. (1994). Child dissociation and the family context. *Journal of Abnormal Child Psychology, 22*, 373-388.

Ogawa, J.R., Sroufe, L.A., Weinfield, N.S., Carlson, E.A., & Egeland, B. (1997). Development and the fragmented self: Longitudinal study of dissociative symptomatology in a nonclinical sample. *Development and Psychopathology, 9*, 855-879.

Plattner, B., Silvermann, M.A., & Redlich, A.D. (2003). Pathways to dissociation: Intrafamilial versus extrafamilial trauma in juvenile delinquents. *Journal of Nervous and Mental Disease, 191*, 781-788.

Putnam, F.W. (1993). Dissociative disorders in children: Behavioral profiles and problem. *Child Abuse and Neglect, 17*, 39-45.

Putnam, F.W. (1997). *Dissociation in children and adolescents: A developmental perspective.* New York: The Guilford Press.

Pynoos, R., Rodriguez, N., Steinberg, A., Stuber, M., & Frederick, C. (1998). *UCLA PTSD index for DSM IV.* Los Angeles: Trauma Psychiatric Services.

Robinson, C.C., Mandleco, B.L., Olsen, S.F., Bancroft-Andrews, C., McNeilly, M. K., & Nelson, L. (1995). Authoritative, authoritarian, and permissive parenting practices: Development of a new measure. *Psychological Reports, 77*, 819-830.

Rossman, B.B.R. & Rea, J.G. (2005). The relation of parenting styles and inconsistencies to adaptive functioning for children in conflictual and violent families. *Journal of Family Violence, 20*, 261-277.

Silberg, J.L. (2000). Fifteen years of dissociation in maltreated children: Where do we go from here? *Child Maltreatment, 5*, 119-136.

Trickett, P.K., Noll, J.G., Reiffman, A., & Putnam, F. (2001). Variants of intrafamilial sexual abuse experience: Implications for short- and long-term development. *Development and Psychopathology, 13*, 1001-1019.

Trickett, P., Duran, L., & Horn, J. (2003). Community violence as it affects child development: Issues of definition. *Clinical Child and Family Psychology Review, 6*, 223-236.

doi:10.1300/J229v07n04_05

Investigating Peri-Traumatic Dissociation Using Hypnosis During a Traumatic Film

Emily A. Holmes, PhD
David A. Oakley, PhD
Ailsa D. P. Stuart, DClinPsy
Chris R. Brewin, PhD

SUMMARY. We investigated the hypothesis that inducing a dissociative response (detachment) in healthy volunteers while they were watching a trauma film would lead to increased numbers of intrusive memories of the film during the following week. Hypnotized participants were given suggestions to dissociate during part of the film, and to watch the rest of

---

Emily A. Holmes is affiliated with the Sub-Department of Clinical Health Psychology, University College London, Gower Street, London, WC1E 6BT, UK and the Department of Psychiatry, University of Oxford, Warneford Hospital, Oxford, OX3 7JX, UK.

David A. Oakley is affiliated with the Hypnosis Unit, Department of Psychology, University College London, Gower Street, London, WC1E 6BT, UK.

Ailsa D. P. Stuart and Chris R. Brewin are affiliated with the Sub-Department of Clinical Health Psychology, University College London, Gower Street, London, WC1E 6BT, UK.

Address correspondence to: Dr. Emily Holmes, Royal Society Dorothy Hodgkin Fellow, University of Oxford, Department of Psychiatry, Warneford Hospital, Oxford, OX3 7JX, UK (E-mail: emily.holmes@psych.ox.ac.uk).

The authors are grateful for the support of Camden and Islington Mental Health and Social Care Trust. Professor Anke Ehlers kindly lent the video.

[Haworth co-indexing entry note]: "Investigating Peri-Traumatic Dissociation Using Hypnosis During a Traumatic Film." Holmes, Emily A. et al. Co-published simultaneously in *Journal of Trauma & Dissociation* (The Haworth Medical Press, an imprint of The Haworth Press, Inc.) Vol. 7, No. 4, 2006, pp. 91-113; and: *Exploring Dissociation: Definitions, Development and Cognitive Correlates* (ed: Anne P. DePrince, and Lisa DeMarni Cromer) The Haworth Medical Press, an imprint of The Haworth Press, Inc., 2006, pp. 91-113. Single or multiple copies of this article are available for a fee from The Haworth Document Delivery Service [1-800-HAWORTH, 9:00 a.m. - 5:00 p.m. (EST). E-mail address: docdelivery@haworthpress.com].

Available online at http://jtd.haworthpress.com
doi:10.1300/J229v07n04_06

the film normally from their own perspective. The order of these conditions, and the section of film watched under the two conditions, were counterbalanced. As predicted, watching the film under both conditions led to increases in dissociation. Explicit suggestions to dissociate were generally effective in inducing higher levels of dissociation. Contrary to prediction, there were no more intrusive memories of sections of the film for which participants had received dissociation suggestions. Implications of our results for views of the relationship between peri-traumatic dissociation and intrusive memories are discussed. doi:10.1300/ J229v07n04_06 *[Article copies available for a fee from The Haworth Document Delivery Service: 1-800-HAWORTH. E-mail address: <docdelivery@haworthpress. com> Website: <http://www.HaworthPress.com> © 2006 by The Haworth Press, Inc. All rights reserved.]*

KEYWORDS. Trauma, hypnosis, intrusive imagery, dissociation, stressful film, PTSD

Dissociation is a response that is thought to protect individuals from experiencing overwhelming emotion. Several cognitive models of posttraumatic stress disorder (PTSD) have suggested that dissociation at the time of trauma may protect against extreme emotions such as fear and horror at that point in time (Brewin & Holmes, 2003). For example, a client with PTSD may report an out-of-body experience or feelings of unreality during the index trauma. Therapists may help the client make sense of such dissociative experiences as an understandable psychological response to trauma particularly perhaps when physical escape is not possible. However, there is now considerable evidence that reports of dissociative reactions during traumatic events are related to an increased risk of posttraumatic stress disorder subsequently developing (Ozer, Best, Lipsey, & Weiss, 2003). These naturalistic studies that rely on retrospective reports have been supplemented by experimental studies in which healthy volunteers watching a traumatic film describe their reactions immediately at the end of the film. Under these conditions, too, higher levels of reported dissociation predict a greater number of intrusive memories of the film in the succeeding week (Holmes, Brewin, & Hennessy, 2004). Using a similar paradigm, the current study attempted to establish the causal role of dissociation in producing post-trauma symptoms by attempting to induce an appropriate dissociative experience hypnotically and then investigating later reactions to a trauma film. Interestingly, although a link is commonly assumed in the literature, it is unclear precisely how dissociation may operate to produce intrusive memories. However, rather than exploring theoretical possibilities for an explanation of the link between the two, the current study attempts to seek further evidence that analogue peri-traumatic dissociation may indeed be associated with a greater number of intrusive memories.

The term 'dissociation' is notoriously complex and has been used in a variety of ways. In their review exploring what is meant by the term 'dissociation' Holmes et al. (2005) distinguished two forms–detachment and compartmentalisation. Post-traumatic stress disorder patients describe both a sense of detachment at the time of the trauma (commonly referred to as peri-traumatic dissociation) and impaired recall of the event, which may correspond better with compartmentalisation. In this study we attempted to manipulate analogue peri-traumatic detachment. However, in the literature described below this distinction has usually not been made thus the term 'dissociation' in the context of trauma can be used as an umbrella term referring to both detachment and compartmentalisation. For further details about this definition and a further development of this model, see Brown (2006, this volume).

To date there have been several studies that have tried to induce dissociation experimentally. Murray (1997) asked participants to try to dissociate while watching a film involving a series of road traffic accidents. Guidelines were provided to help them do this, and participants were asked to practise strategies such as staring at a spot on the wall, staring into a mirror, or imagining that they were watching themselves from an external vantage point. There was no specific check that participants in this condition experienced more dissociative symptoms while watching the film. They rated themselves as moderately able to follow these instructions, but were not as successful as participants in other groups following different instructions to perform other tasks. Participants instructed to dissociate did not experience more intrusive memories involving the film in the following week than did those in a control condition.

Holmes et al. (2004) conducted a similar experiment using the same trauma film. They based their approach on a review of methods of inducing concurrent dissociation (Leonard, Telch, & Harrington, 1999), which suggested that prolonged staring at a small dot was likely to be effective. To ensure that participants were able to comply with the task, an initial screening phase was devised to eliminate those who were unable to dissociate using this method. The success of the manipulation was confirmed using a self-report measure of state dissociation, but again participants in this group did not experience more intrusive memories of a trauma film than those in a control group. Moreover, the self-report measure of dissociation did not correlate with drops in heart rate, a physiological measure that may also be an index of dissociation (Griffin, Resick, & Mechanic, 1997).

Hypnosis is becoming more widely accepted as a cognitive tool in psychological and neuropsychological research (Oakley, 2006, Raz & Shapriro, 2002) and we have recently begun to explore hypnotically suggested dissociative experiences as a potentially useful experimental analogue for traumatic dissociation. Suggestion in hypnosis has been used in experimental settings to create subjectively compelling, but reversible, experiences of amnesia for autobiographical episodes (Barnier, McConkey & Wright, 2004), emotional numbing (Bryant, 2005), gender change (Burn, Barnier & McConkey, 2003), functional blindness (Bryant & McConkey, 1999), auditory hallucinations (Szechtman, Woody, Bowers & Nahmias, 1998), non-veridical colour processing (Kosslyn, Thompson, Costantini-Ferrando, Alpert & Spiegel, 2000), functional pain (Derbyshire, Whalley, Stenger & Oakley, 2004), involuntary movement (Blakemore, Oakley & Frith, 2003; Haggard, Cartledge, Dafydd & Oakley, 2004) and functional paralysis (Halligan, Athwal, Oakley & Frackowiak, 2000). A number of these studies have also involved neuroimaging and have found that the suggested phenomena are accompanied by congruent changes in activation in brain areas that would normally be involved in mediating the processes affected by the hypnotic suggestion (Blakemore et al., 2003; Derbyshire et al., 2004; Halligan et al., 2000; Kosslyn et al., 2000; Szechtman et al., 1998). This is consistent with the subjectively 'as-real' nature of hypnotically induced experiential changes. The same patterns of brain activity were not seen, however, when individuals were asked to imagine the same subjective events (Kosslyn et al., 2000) even when this was carried out in hypnosis (Derbyshire et al., 2004; Szechtman et al., 1998) or when hypnotised participants were instructed to simulate the hypnotically suggested effect (Ward, Oakley, Frackowiak & Halligan, 2003).

A common theme in the studies that have used hypnosis as an experimental tool is that the suggested effects are more strongly produced in individuals who are rated as medium to high in hypnotic susceptibility. It is interesting in this regard that there is convergent evidence that post-traumatic stress disorder and its symptoms are associated with higher levels of hypnotizability (Bryant, Guthrie, Moulds, Nixon & Felmingham, 2003). This raises the possibility of common underlying mechanisms between symptoms seen in post-traumatic stress disorder and comparable phenomena produced by suggestion in hypnosis. A similar case has been made for hypnotic phenomena and functional clinical symptoms (Oakley, 1999) with some supporting neuroimaging evidence for commonality in mechanism in the case of 'hysterical' (conversion disorder) limb paralysis and the corresponding hypnotically-produced paralysis (Halligan et al., 2000).

On the strength of this emerging evidence of the efficacy of hypnosis as an experimental tool we have recently adopted a similar approach to investigate the impact on intrusive images of experimentally induced somatoform dissociation (tonic immobility) during a stressful film (Hagenaars, van Minnen, Holmes, Brewin & Hoogduin, 2006). Hypnotic suggestions were used to create catalepsy–that is to immobilize participants while viewing the film. This manipulation was designed to mimic the 'freezing' response that can be reported by people during a traumatic event (Nijenhuis, Van Engen, Kusters, & Van der Hart, 2001). Two comparison conditions were used, an 'intentional no movement' group, where participants were instructed to intentionally keep still but did not use hypnotic suggestion to create a cataleptic state, and a control group who were told they could sit and move as they wished while viewing the film. The results showed that the catalepsy condition proved an effective way of provoking somatoform dissociation. However, both experimental task conditions increased the number of intrusive images of the film compared to the control condition. No difference was found in intrusions between dissociation-related immobility and voluntary immobility. This suggests that it is unlikely that somatoform dissociation *per se* is responsible for an increase in trauma film images, but the immobility itself may have been an active ingredient.

To summarise, several attempts have now been made to induce dissociation experimentally. Although there have been some positive results in terms of changes on self-report measures, none has succeeded in bringing about a change in posttraumatic symptomatology such as the frequency of intrusive memories or has been able to show that dissociative aspects accounted for this. The current experiment again used hypnotic suggestion but with the intention of reproducing aspects of peri-traumatic dissociation other than the immobility or 'freezing' already investigated by Hagenaars et al. (2006). This raises the persistent problem in analogue studies of defining the target phenomenon. As discussed previously, Holmes et al. (2005) have divided the term 'dissociation' into two forms–detachment and compartmentalisation. In this study we attempted to manipulate the experience of detachment as an analogue for peri-traumatic dissociation.

A within-subjects design was used whereby participants viewed a traumatic film while hypnotised. Some sections of the film were viewed following suggestions intended to generate peri-traumatic dissociation and other sections were viewed without such suggestions (Suggested Dissociation versus Control condition). As well as testing the ability of suggested dissociation to bring about appropriate changes in self-report measures, we also assessed whether there would be a concomitant change in peri-traumatic distress and in the experience of intrusive memories.

Consistent with the theory that peri-traumatic dissociation protects individuals at the time from overwhelming emotion but increases later vulnerability to PTSD, we predicted that:

1. State dissociation (for details see the Measures section) will increase as a result of viewing the film under either condition compared to a baseline (pre-film).
2. Participants will report higher levels of state dissociation in the Suggested Dissociation condition compared to the Control condition.
3. Participants will report lower levels of peri-traumatic distress in the Suggested Dissociation condition compared to the Control condition.
4. Participants will report more intrusive images during the week after the film in the Suggested Dissociation condition compared to the Control condition.

METHOD

Design

This study used a within-subjects design that involved viewing a film showing distressing scenes from road traffic accidents. The film was divided into two sections each of which was viewed by hypnotised participants under one of two conditions: (1) following suggestions designed to evoke dissociative experiences (Suggested Dissociation condition) and (2) under the same viewing conditions but without suggestions for dissociation (Control condition). The order of these two viewing conditions and the order of presentation of the two film sections were independently counterbalanced. Measures of distress and state dissociation were collected after both sections of the film. Participants also recorded their experience of intrusions from the film in a diary for 1 week after the viewing and then returned for a follow-up session.

Participants

Ethical approval for this study was granted by the Joint UCL/UCLH Committees on the Ethics of Human Research, Study Number 01/0063. All participants gave their informed consent to taking part in the research. Recruitment took place from a volunteer database of seventy-three students from the Departments of Psychology and Medicine at University College London who had been previously categorised as highly or very highly hypnotisable (scoring 8 or more out of 12) on the Harvard Group Scale of Hypnotic Susceptibility: Form A (HGSHS:A; Shor & Orne, 1962). The recruitment material included information about the traumatic film, in particular that it contained graphic scenes of the aftermath of road traffic accidents that could be involuntarily remembered afterwards. All participants confirmed in writing that they had not previously received treatment for a mental health problem in order to ensure informed consent. Of the 73 potential participants contacted by one email message (sent blind to other recipients), seventeen agreed to take part in the current experiment (12 male and 5 female) and received a small payment. Due to missing data for one participant, the final results presented are based on 16 participants. The mean age of those who volunteered was 20.31 ($SD = 0.95$, range 19-22). Their mean hypnotic susceptibility score was 9.25, $SD = 1.00$, range 8-11) and mean trait dissociation (DES-II) score was 10.30 ($SD = 12.33$). All participants were tested singly.

Materials

Trauma video film. The 12.5 minutes of video film material used here comprised real-life scenes from the aftermath of five different road traffic accidents in Germany (compiled by Steil, 1996, used previously for example by Murray, 1997; Halligan, Clark, & Ehlers, 2002; Holmes et al., 2004; Stuart et al., 2006). The film included: victims being extracted from wreckage by emergency services personnel, injured victims screaming, body parts amongst wreckage and bodies being transferred to coffins. Previous studies (Holmes et al., 2004) have collected information about the content of intrusive images arising from this film, which allowed each intrusion to be located to a particular scene (intrusion sequence). This information from approximately 200 participants was used by Stuart et al. (2006) to calculate the average number intrusions that arose from each of the five scenes. Instead of dividing the film in terms of time (which could result in scenes with different relative intrusiveness) the film was divided into two (counterbalanced) sections that were expected to generate similar amounts of intrusions, as in Stuart et al. (2006).

Measures

Hypnotic susceptibility. The *Harvard Group Scale of Hypnotic Susceptibility. Form A (HGSHS:A*; Shor & Orne, 1962) is administered to groups of participants and consists of a hypnotic induction procedure followed by 12 standard suggestions (categorised as 'ideo-motor,' 'challenge' and 'cognitive') intended to create clearly defined subjective experiences with accompanying behavioural changes that are experienced as being involuntary and effortless. Responses to each of these suggestions are scored on a pass (1) or fail (0) basis giving a range of possible scores from 0 to 12. Individuals scoring 11-12 are categorised as 'very highly hypnotizable' (5-7% of the normal population) and those scoring 8-10 as 'highly hypnotizable' (17-34%) (Barnier & McConkey, 2004). The HGSHS:A used to create the database from which participants were recruited for this study was delivered by audiotape.

Trait Dissociation. The *Dissociative Experiences Scale–Revised version (DES-II*; Carlson & Putnam, 1993) is a 28-item scale on which participants indicate the percentage of time they have a given dissociative experience in daily life, from 0% (never) to 100% (always). It provides a trait type measure of dissociative experiences.

State Dissociation. Three measures were used to assess various aspects of dissociative experiences during the experiment. The first was a pre-post measure of state dissociation that has been used in previous experimental studies (e.g., Holmes et al., 2004). The second measure is a widely used clinical measure to assess peri-traumatic dissociation, relying on retrospective report experience during trauma. The third measure consisted of individually tailored visual analogue scale ratings related to suggestions given in the Suggested Dissociation condition of this experiment. Thus the first measure uses a difference score whereas the second two measures yield single scores.

1. The 19 subject-rated items from the *Clinician Administered Dissociative States Scale (referred to here as the DSS;* Bremner et al., 1998) were used as a repeated measure of state dissociation to assess

relevant symptom areas including depersonalization and derealization. Items are rated on a 5-point scale anchored with 0 (not at all) and 4 (extremely). A sample item is "Do things appear to be moving in slow motion." The 19 items have satisfactory reliability (Cronbach's alpha = .94; Bremner et al., 1998).

2. The *Peritraumatic Dissociative Experiences Questionnaire (PDEQ*; Marmar, Weiss, & Metzler, 1997) is a measure of dissociative symptoms experienced at the time of trauma. The 10 items on this questionnaire are rated on a 5-point scale. As it asks participants about their experiences of dissociation *during* a particular time period it is particularly useful to use in a within-subjects design where two time periods are being compared.

3. Three *Visual Analogue Scales (VAS)* were used to rate specific dissociative experiences during the viewing of the film in the context of the suggestions given in the Suggested Dissociation condition. Participants were asked to indicate by making a mark on a 100mm line how strongly they felt the experience (i) of observing themselves looking at the film, (ii) as if viewing the film was happening to someone else, and (iii) of world around them being strange and unreal. The ends of the lines for each scale were anchored with 'I did not get that feeling at all' (0) and 'The feeling was very strong indeed' (100).

Distress. Participants rated their distress associated with viewing the film on an 11-point scale anchored with 0 'not at all distressed' and 10 'extremely distressed.'

Intrusions. Participants were instructed in how to use a tabular *Intrusion Diary* in which they were asked to record any intrusive images from the film for the 7 days following viewing it (as in Holmes et al., 2004). Each day was divided into four periods: morning, afternoon, evening and night. Intrusions were defined as 'intrusive memories of the film that suddenly pop into mind spontaneously' and not 'times when you deliberately think about it or mull over it.' The content of each intrusion experienced was also recorded so that the intrusions could later be identified as coming from a particular section of the film (for more details of this method see also Stuart, Holmes & Brewin, 2006). For example, if the participant described an intrusive image of 'a fireman carrying a baby' this event only occurred at one point in the film, this image could be retrospectively matched according to within-subjects condition (i.e., what the participant had been doing at the time of encoding). Thus the number of intrusions was later calculated for each within-subjects condition. Participants were asked to carry the diary with them and fill in the appropriate sections at regular times during the day (divided into morning, afternoon and evening). They were also asked to set aside a specific time at the end of the day to complete the diary, even if they had had no intrusions, in which case they should enter a zero in the number box.

At the follow-up session, a *Diary Compliance Rating* was taken by asking participants to rate the truthfulness of the statement 'I have often been unable (or forgotten) to record my intrusions in the diary' (Davies & Clark, 1998). The response scale was anchored with 0 (*not at all true*) to 10 (*completely true*), hence low scores indicate good compliance.

Procedure

After providing their informed consent to take part in the study, participants provided information about their age and completed the DES-II and DSS (baseline administration) questionnaire measures. Participants then sat in a chair approximately 1m from the television screen facing directly towards it throughout the experimental procedures. The two experimenters sat outside the participant's line of sight, with Experimenter 2 to their right and Experimenter 1 to their far left. Experimenter 2 used a standardised protocol to explore the participant's previous experiences of hypnosis, to personalise the induction script for them and to identify their unique 'Special Place' (Oakley, Deeley, & Halligan 2006).

Experimenter 2 then used the personalised standard induction script commencing with the participant's eyes closed, followed by instructions and suggestions for regular breathing and muscle relaxation, descent imagery and experience of their 'Special Place.' Half the participants were then exposed to the Suggested Dissociation condition while viewing one section of the film and then to the Control condition while viewing the other section. The order of these conditions was reversed for the other participants. It is noted that participants remained hypnotized during both conditions. Thus, the two within-subjects conditions were determined according to the dissociation suggestions or the control condition instructions.

For the Suggested Dissociation condition suggestions were given to create the subjective experience while they were viewing the film section of being disconnected from their body ('looking at the screen but seeing it from a different perspective as though you are viewing it from outside your own body–from a different point of view. . . '); of feeling as if they were 'someone else' ('. . . as though you were another person . . . being aware of the screen and being aware of yourself watching it') and that the world around them was strange and unreal ('. . . everything around you seeming strange and unreal as though you were somehow another person in a strange place.'). Additional suggestions were included to ensure that they continued to attend to the film while having these experiences ('When you open your eyes [you will] continue to have those feelings as you watch what is shown on the screen–being fully aware of the events taking place. . . . '). These suggestions were intended to emulate dissociative peri-traumatic experiences of detachment commonly reported in PTSD.

Once the dissociation suggestions had been given participants were told they would 'Continue to have these feelings for the whole time you watch the film until you are given different instructions. Stay as hypnotized as you are now, open your eyes and watch the film.' At the end of the Suggested Dissociation condition the participant was asked by Experimenter 2 to shut their eyes and suggestions were given that they were 'returning to normal feelings, experiencing the world from your own perspective–everything feeling as real and normal as it should.' When the participant indicated that this has occurred they were asked to return to their Special Place experience.

For the Control condition participants were told that when they opened their eyes they would watch the film as they normally would 'from your own perspective' and then 'Stay as hypnotized as you are now, open your eyes and watch the film.' No reference was made to being 'relaxed' or feeling 'normal' while watching the film. At the end of the Control condition viewing the participant was asked to return to their special place experience. For the full hypnotic script for each condition, please see Appendix 1.

For all participants there was a break of approximately two minutes between the two viewings of the two counterbalanced sections of the film during which they remained hypnotized and experiencing their Special Place. Once testing under both conditions was complete all hypnotic suggestions were removed and hypnosis was terminated. The rating of distress when viewing the film, the DSS, the PDEQ, and the VAS ratings of dissociative experiences were then recorded separately for both viewings of the film. After finishing both conditions, participants were instructed in how to complete the intrusion diaries. One week later there was a follow-up session at which participants returned their intrusion diaries and rated their diary compliance. Participants were debriefed and thanked for their participation. In our clinical opinion, no participant displayed a significant level of distress at the follow-up session. Following ethical guidelines a procedure was in place should participants subsequently wish to make contact with the experimenters, but none did so.

RESULTS

The data analysis software used was SPSS version 13 for Windows.

Measures of State Dissociation

DSS. In order to examine whether, as predicted, the experience of dissociation would increase as a result of viewing the film under either condition as compared to baseline (pre-film), we examined only the scores from baseline to the end of the first condition. Due to the counter-balanced order of presentation, for half of the participants the first condition was Suggested Dissociation and for half the Control condition. Paired sample *t*-tests were used on the data shown in Table 1. There was a significant increase in state dissociation from baseline in the Suggested Dissociation condition, $t(8) = 8.16$, $p < .001$, mean change = 22.56 ($SD = 8.29$), $d = 4.84$ indicating a large effect size. There was also a significant increase in the Control condition, $t(6) = 5.17$, $p = .002$, mean change = 9.29 ($SD = 4.75$), $d = 3.12$ indicating a large effect size.

In order to examine whether changes in state dissociation were significantly greater in the Suggested Dissociation than in the Control condition, change scores were computed by subtracting the DSS score before each condition from the DSS score after that condition. The data were entered into a 2 (Experimental condition: Suggested Dissociation versus Control Condition) × 2 (Order: Suggested Dissociation first versus Control Condition first) mixed model ANOVA. Experimental condition was a repeated measures factor and Order a between-subjects factor. There was a significant main effect of Experimental condition on change in dissociation, $F(1,14) = 32.65$, $p < .001$, partial eta squared = 0.70, indicating a large effect size. There was a significant main effect of Order, $F(1,14) = 1.52$, $p = .024$, partial eta squared = 0.50, indicating a large effect size. There was also a significant interaction between Experimental condition and Order, $F(1,14) = 37.45$, $p = .002$, partial eta squared = 0.73, again indicating a large effect size.

This interaction was decomposed by using two paired sample t-tests to examine the effect of Experimental condition on change in state dissociation for each of the two Orders. As shown in Table 1, when Suggested Dissociation was followed by the Control condition, there was a

TABLE 1. Mean DSS scores across three time points for both orders of experimental condition.

	Order 1 (N = 7)			Order 2 (N = 9)		
	Baseline	Control condition	Suggested Dissociation condition	Baseline	Suggested Dissociation condition	Control condition
DSS score mean (SD)	1.71 (2.98)	11.00 (5.07)	18.86 (11.39)	2.89 (4.68)	25.44 (9.99)	6.33 (4.06)

significant difference in state dissociation change between the experimental conditions, $t(8) = 8.33$, $p < .001$, $d = 5.29$, with mean change scores in line with predictions, $+22.56$ ($SD = 8.29$) vs. -19.00 (7.86). However, when the Control condition was first no significant difference was found, $t(6) = 0.30$, $p = .77$, $d = 0.30$, equivalent mean change scores $= 7.86$ ($SD = 9.67$) vs 9.29 ($SD = 4.75$). Thus with respect to the initial hypotheses, our results indicate that Suggested Dissociation led to a greater increase in state dissociation as measured by the DSS than the Control condition but that this increase was significant only when Suggested Dissociation came first in the experimental order.

PDEQ. A similar mixed-model analysis on retrospective ratings of dissociative experiences during the film indicated a significant main effect of Experimental condition on PDEQ scores, $F(1,14) = 25.41$, $p < .001$, partial eta squared $= 0.65$, indicating a large effect size. There was no significant main effect of Order, $F(1,14) = 0.11$, $p = .75$, and no significant interaction between Experimental condition and Order, $F(1,14) = 0.89$, $p = .36$. The mean overall PDEQ score for the Suggested Dissociation condition was 24.37 ($SD = 6.90$) and for the Control condition was 15.56 ($SD = 4.91$).

VAS. Participant ratings of the three dimensions of dissociative experience (related to the experimental suggestions) in the Suggested Dissociation and Control conditions are shown in Table 2. A comparison of scores using related t tests revealed significant differences in the predicted direction between conditions on each of the three ratings. Order effects were investigated using mixed-model ANOVAs but there were no main effects of order or condition by order interactions except for a weak main effect of order on the extent participants felt they were seeing themselves from outside of their own body, $F(1,14) = 4.80$, $p = .046$, partial eta squared $= .25$.

TABLE 2. The additional ratings of dissociative experience in each experimental condition.

Rating of dissociative experience	Suggested Dissociation condition Mean (SD)	Control condition Mean (SD)	$t(15)$
Outside your body	51.18 (25.01)	9.94 (14.84)	7.32*
Feeling as if you were someone else	47.94 (25.22)	16.41 (23.98)	5.53*
Other people and objects feeling strange and unreal	52.12 (31.00)	10.47 (15.65)	5.76*

*p < .001

Distress Ratings

It was predicted that participants in the Suggested Dissociation condition, compared to the control condition, would report the lower levels of peri-traumatic distress. In line with this prediction, there was significant difference in the amount of distress experienced during the Suggested Dissociation condition ($M = 4.38$, $SD = 2.25$) compared to the control condition ($M = 6.31$, $SD = 1.96$), $t(15) = 3.18$, $p = .006$, $d = .98$. Possible order effects were explored using mixed-model ANOVAs, but there was no significant effect of order and no condition by order interaction.

Intrusive Images of the Film

Consistent with previous studies, the mean level of diary compliance was 2.00 ($SD = 1.37$), indicating that participants had recorded most of their intrusions in the diary. Forty-four intrusive images were recorded. Of these images, there were six which we were unable to identify within the film. The remaining images corresponded to a clear moment within the traumatic film (e.g., a fireman carrying a baby), which enabled us to calculate how many of each participant's intrusions came from each condition (c.f. Stuart et al., 2005).

The mean number of images from the Suggested Dissociation condition was 0.94 ($SD = 1.00$) while the mean number of images from the Control condition was 1.69 ($SD = 1.54$). These data were entered into a 2 (Experimental condition: Suggested Dissociation versus Control) × 2 (Order: Suggested Dissociation condition first versus Control condition first) mixed model ANOVA. There were no significant effects of Experimental condition, $F(1,14) = 3.13$, $MSE = 1.46$, $p = 0.098$, partial eta squared = 0.18, or Order F (1,14) = 2.17, MSE = 1.85, p = 0.16, partial eta squared = 0.13. Inspection of F values however, given the small sample size, indicates that future studies with better power might usefully explore this issue. The interaction was also non-significant, F (1,14) = 0.08, p = .93. Since the interaction was non-significant, helpful comments by reviewers suggested that we further examine the intrusion data using a paired sample t-test for the number of intrusions between condition. The results of this again hint towards a trend in the *opposite* direction to that predicted, that mean value indicate the suggested dissociation condition may have been associated with fewer (rather than more) intrusive images, t (15) = 1.82, p = .091, d = 0.49. However, given the small sample size and power of the study any conclusions drawn must be tentative.

Qualitative Findings

Participants offered some comments describing their experience of Suggested Dissociation. These are included here to provide some qualitative information about the experience of the manipulation. The themes contained in the suggestions we gave our participants of being disconnected from their body, as if they were someone else and in a world that had become strange and unreal are all clearly reflected along with some embellishments of their own.

Feelings of detachment were frequently mentioned: 'I felt really strange–like the lights were on but nobody was in. I felt as though I wasn't me. I felt as though I was viewing it from outside.'; 'It felt weird, you are watching it but not as yourself–as someone else.'; 'Physically I felt different–I was watching the film separately from my body.' For some the experiences were accompanied by distortions of body image: 'The whole experience felt unreal, as if I wasn't there. . . . also my feet felt really big–what was that all about?'; 'I felt really tall as though I was above my body.' For others the sense of altered viewing location was particularly noticeable: 'It was too strange–I've never felt anything like it.–I was crouched on the small filing cabinet across the way [over to the left of him].'; 'I kinda thought I was over there [points to his right] looking at you guys. But I thought it was weird; I'm not there I'm in the chair! . . . I was watching someone else but someone else was wearing my clothes.'; 'I could see myself sitting to my right . . . I could sense myself watching myself from the other view and I could see what I was watching.' Their comments also reflected the reduced distress they experienced when watching in the Suggested Dissociation condition:

'I felt less involved and interested than [in] the other film. I was watching and feeling it should be a lot more distressing'; 'It didn't seem half as bad, the people in it were just actors and it didn't seem half as gruesome.'

DISCUSSION

To our knowledge this is the first study to attempt to induce a dissociative state of detachment using hypnosis, comparing responses in a within-subjects design to a control condition in which participants were hypnotized but not given dissociation suggestions. The measure of state dissociation (DSS) that was taken before as well as after the experimental manipulations confirmed our first prediction, that watching the trauma video in the control condition would be associated with spontaneous dissociation. Ratings taken after film viewings using a standardized (and clinically used) measure of peri-traumatic dissociation as well as individual rating scales confirmed our second and third predictions that participants would report higher levels of dissociative experiences and less distress in the Suggested Dissociation condition. Further analysis of the DSS data revealed a more complex picture, however. In particular, the experimental manipulation did not appear to be so effective when the Suggested Dissociation condition came second (Order 1), as participants tended to respond more strongly with spontaneous dissociative experiences to watching the film during the first, Control, condition. When the Suggested Dissociation condition came first (Order 2), however, spontaneous dissociation in the Control condition appeared less marked and the difference in dissociation between the conditions was clear-cut.

It is important to emphasize that if the spontaneous dissociation elicited by the trauma film had not been entered into the DSS analysis it is likely that there would have been significant differences between the conditions in Order 1 also. Another factor to take into account is that the power to detect differences between conditions in this study was in any case low because of the relatively small numbers of participants. Overall, therefore, the formal measures employed here have provided promising evidence that dissociative experiences can be effectively manipulated by hypnotic suggestion. The effectiveness of the manipulation was also underscored by comments offered by participants describing their experience of Suggested Dissociation (see the Results section on Qualitative Findings). However, there are some limitations that are addressed below.

We feel that the study reported here merits replication and extension. In future studies using within-subjects designs of this sort it should be borne in mind, however, that data acquired retrospectively on completion of the experiment may be subject to demand characteristics, and measures should be included at the beginning and end of each condition wherever possible. As well as the small sample size there are several other methodological limitations to this study which means interpretations drawn should be made with caution. Although participants all confirmed that they had not attended mental health services in the past, this does not rule out the possibility that they may have experienced trauma, and as a result PTSD, even if only at a sub-clinical level. In line with previous experimental work attempting to investigate the impact of peri-traumatic dissociation on analogue PTSD symptoms (e.g., Holmes et al., 2004; Murray, 1997; Stuart et al., 2006), we have focussed on intrusive images of the trauma. Methodologically this allows us to use this type of within-subject design and manipulate processing during particular sequences of analogue trauma. Perhaps future methodological innovations might develop ways in which avoidance or hyperarousal could be assessed within this type of design. Future studies may also benefit from examining different types of trauma films (e.g., Orsillo, Plumb, Luterek, & Roessner, 2004). Dissociation is a complex construct and we used three measures of state dissociation to assess this and make comparable to other research: a repeated measure as used in previous experimental paradigms, a clinical measure of retrospective report, as well as tailored rating scales for the hypnotic suggestions. However, it is possible that the use of multiple ANOVAs increased family wise error rates.

Consistent with all previous attempts to induce dissociation experimentally (Hagenaars et al., 2006; Holmes et al., 2004, Exp. 1; Murray, 1997), we did not succeed in significantly influencing the number of intrusive memories of the trauma film participants recorded in their diaries. Indeed, mean values appeared in the opposite value to that predicted, that is the Suggested Dissociation condition had a smaller mean number of images than the Control condition. These results contrast with data indicating that both trait dissociation (Holmes et al., 2004; Murray, 1997), and spontaneous state dissociation (Holmes et al., 2004, Experiments 1 and 2) are correlated with increased levels of subsequent intrusions. One possibility is that attempts to experimentally manipulate dissociation have mostly been limited to those aspects that represent detachment, to use the distinction employed by Holmes et al. (2005). For an exception see Hagenaars et al. (2006) who manipulated catalepsy-pseudo-paralysis may be more akin to compartmentalization. An alternative approach would be to manipulate other features of dissociation that reflect other aspects of compartmentalization, such as partial amnesia. This could be done in a hypnotic context for example by eliciting selective or partial amnesia for the viewing experience and the content of the video with suggestions designed to produce the sort of memory distortions and losses typically reported in PTSD. It may be that the experience of detachment serves the protective function of reducing the distress experienced at the time of the trauma but it may be compartmentalization of memory functions that leads to later intrusions. While Holmes et al. (2005) highlight there are two forms of 'dissociation'–detachment and compartmentalization–both these forms further subdivide. In this study we attempted to manipulate those aspects of analogue peri-traumatic detachment highlighted in the hypnotic suggestions. In future work on analogue trauma we may need to more precisely manipulate, and use outcome measures which tap into these various forms of 'dissociation.'

A second possible explanation for the lack of a significant difference in intrusions between the two conditions is that spontaneous dissociation in the Control condition had produced a ceiling effect so that increasing dissociation still further had no additional influence on subsequent intrusions. One way of testing this possibility would be to use hypnotic suggestion to *reduce* the level of dissociation in the experimental condition using the reverse of the suggestions used in the present study to inhibit spontaneous dissociation whilst viewing a trauma film.

A third possibility is that though there are similarities between reports of spontaneous and the suggested dissociative experiences used here there may nevertheless be important differences between the two. As we reviewed in the introduction, there is increasing evidence of functional convergence between hypnotically suggested phenomena and their more naturally occurring counterparts, in many instances the similarities are supported by evidence from neuroimaging. It would be interesting in the light of this to compare brain activations in spontaneous and hypnotically suggested dissociative states using both neutral and trauma film viewing. We would anticipate very similar patterns of brain activation in the hypnotically suggested and the spontaneous dissociation conditions. However any differences might give a clue as to what is perhaps missing from hypnotically suggested dissociation but is present in spontaneous dissociation and this in turn may explain the relative lack of effect of hypnotically suggested dissociation (detachment) on subsequent intrusions.

Hypnotically suggested dissociation, in common with hypnotic phenomena generally, appears to occur involuntarily and effortlessly–there were no reports from our participants that they had to make any conscious effort to produce the suggested experiences. However this may not be the case in earlier studies that used other strategies to generate analogue dissociative states. It may be important that individuals in those experiments had to devote effort and attention to the instructions they have been given to dissociate. This requirement may alter the conditions necessary for the development of intrusions. It would be interesting to take a group of people who regularly use dissociation as a coping strategy and ask them to utilize this when watching the film. Another possibility is that dissociation is only associated with later intrusions when it occurs spontaneously, rather than as a deliberate coping strategy or, as in our study, as a suggested state. As in previous studies, we found that participants watching the film reported some dissociative reactions even when they had not been given any instructions to do so. Spontaneous dissociation may, for instance, be a more direct reflection of loss of control or other processes that are linked to intrusion development. Future studies could profitably question participants exhibiting spontaneous dissociation to determine whether this was a voluntary or involuntary reaction.

REFERENCES

Barnier, A.J., & McConkey, K.M. (2004). Defining and identifying the highly hypnotizable person. In M. Heap, R.J. Brown, & D. A. Oakley (Eds.), *The highly hypnotizable person: Theoretical, experimental and clinical issues* (pp. 30-60). London: Routledge.

Barnier, A.J., McConkey, K.M., & Wright, J. (2004). Posthypnotic amnesia for autobiographical episodes: Influencing memory accessibility and quality. *International Journal of Clinical and Experimental Hypnosis, 52*, 260-279.

Blakemore, S-J., Oakley, D.A., & Frith, C.D. (2003). Delusions of alien control in the normal brain. *Neuropsychologia, 41*, 1058-1067.

Bremner, J.D., Krystal, J.H., Putnam, F.W., Southwick, S.M., Marmar, C.R., Charney, D.S., et al. (1998). Measurement of dissociative states with the clinician-administered dissociative states scales (CADSS). *Journal of Traumatic Stress, 11*, 125-136.

Brown, R.J. (2006). Different types of "dissociation" have different psychological mechanisms. *Journal of Trauma and Dissociation, 7*(4), 7-28.

Bryant, R.A. (2005). Hypnotic emotional numbing: A study of implicit emotion. *International Journal of Clinical and Experimental Hypnosis, 53*, 26-36.

Bryant, R.A., Guthrie, R.M., Moulds, M.L., Nixon, R.D.V. & Felmingham, K. (2003). Hypnotizability and posttraumatic stress disorder. *International Journal of Clinical and Experimental Hypnosis, 51*, 382-389.

Bryant, R.A. & McConkey, K.M. (1999). Functional blindness: A construction of cognitive and social influences. *Cognitive Neuropsychiatry, 4*, 227-241.

Burn, C., Barnier, A.J., & Mc Conkey, K.M. (2001). Information processing during hypnotically suggested sex change. *International Journal of Clinical and Experimental Hypnosis, 49*, 231-242.

Carlson, E.B. & Putnam, F.W. (1993). An update on the dissociative experience scale. *Dissociation: Progress in the Dissociative Disorders, 6*, 16-27.

Derbyshire, S.W.G., Whalley, M.G., Stenger, V.A., & Oakley, D.A. (2005). Cerebral activation during hypnotically induced and imagined pain. *NeuroImage, 23*, 392-401.

Griffin, M.G., Resick, P., & Mechanic, M. (1997). Objective assessment of peritraumatic dissociation: Psychophysiological indicators. *American Journal of Psychiatry, 154*, 1081-1088.

Hagenaars, M.A., van Minnen, A., Holmes, E.A., Brewin, C.R., & Hoogduin, K. (2006). The effect of peritraumatic somatoform dissociation on intrusion development after trauma. *Manuscript in preparation.*

Haggard, P., Cartledge, P., Dafydd, M. & Oakley, D.A. (2004). Anomalous control: When 'free-will' is not conscious. *Consciousness & Cognition, 13*, 646-654.

Halligan, P.W., Athwal, B.S., Oakley, D.A., & Frackowiak, R.S.J. (2000). The functional anatomy of a hypnotic paralysis: Implications for conversion hysteria. *The Lancet, 355*, 986-987.

Halligan, S.L., Clark, D.M., & Ehlers, A. (2002). Cognitive processing, memory, and the development of PTSD symptoms: Two experimental analogue studies. *Journal of Behavior Therapy and Experimental Psychiatry, 33*(2), 73-89.

Holmes, E.A., Brewin, C.R., & Hennessy, R.G. (2004). Trauma films, information processing, and intrusive memory development. *Journal of Experimental Psychology: General, 133*, 3-22.

Holmes, E.A., Brown, R.J., Mansell, W., Fearon, R.P., Hunter, E.C.M., Frasquilho, F., & Oakley, D. (2005). Are there two qualitatively distinct forms of dissociation? A review and some clinical implications. *Clinical Psychology Review, 25*, 1-23.

Kosslyn, S.M., Thompson, W.L., Costantini-Ferrando, M.F., Alpert N.M., & Spiegel, D. (2000). Hypnotic visual illusion alters color processing in the brain. *American Journal of Psychiatry, 157*, 1279-1284.

Leonard, K.N., Telch, M.J., & Harrington, P.J. (1999). Dissociation in the laboratory: A comparison of strategies. *Behaviour Research and Therapy, 37*, 49-61.

Murray, J. (1997). The role of dissociation in the development and maintenance of post-traumatic stress disorder. Unpublished doctoral dissertation, Oxford University.

Nijenhuis, E.R.S., Van Engen, A., Kusters, I., & Van der Hart, O. (2001). Peritraumatic somatoform and psychological dissociation in relation to recall of childhood sexual abuse. *Journal of Trauma and Dissociation, 2*, 48-68.

Oakley, D.A. (1999). Hypnosis and conversion hysteria: A unifying model. *Cognitive Neuropsychiatry, 4*, 243-265.

Oakley, D.A. (2006). Hypnosis as a tool in research: Experimental psychopathology. *Contemporary Hypnosis, 23*(1), 3-14.

Oakley, D.A., Deeley, Q., & Halligan, P.W. (2006). Hypnotic depth and response to suggestion under standardised conditions and during fMRI scanning. Manuscript under revision.

Raz, A. & Shapiro, T. (2002). Hypnosis and neuroscience: A cross talk between clinical and cognitive research. *Archives of General Psychiatry, 59*, 85-90.

Stuart, A., Holmes, E.A., & Brewin, C.R. (2006). The influence of a visuospatial grounding task on intrusive images of a traumatic film. *Behaviour Research and Therapy, 44*, 611-619.

Szechtman, H., Woody, E., Bowers, K.S., & Nahmias, C. (1998). Where the imaginal appears real: A positron emission tomography study of auditory hallucinations. *Proceedings of the National Academy of Sciences, 95*, 1956-1960.

Orsillo, S.M., Batten, S.V., Plumb, J.C., Luterek, J.A., & Roessner, B.M. (2004). An experimental study of emotional responding in women with posttraumatic stress disorder related to interpersonal violence. *Journal of Traumatic Stress, 17*, 241-248.

Ozer, E.J., Best, S.R., Lipsey, T.L., & Weiss, D.S. (2003). Predictors of posttraumatic stress disorder and symptoms in adults: A meta-analysis. *Psychological Bulletin, 129*, 52-73.

Ward, N.S., Oakley, D.A., Frackowiak, R.S.J., & Halligan, P.W. (2003). Differential brain activations during intentionally simulated and subjectively experienced paralysis. *Cognitive Neuropsychiatry, 8*, 295-312.

doi:10.1300/J229v07n04_06

APPENDIX 1

Scripts used for (i) Control condition (ii) Suggested dissociation condition.

i. Script for Control Condition

'Stay as hypnotized as you are now with your eyes closed–imagine that you are looking at a television screen–begin to have the experience of the screen in front of you. Watching it normally from your own perspective. *[Pause. Participant is asked to signal with a head nod when this has been achieved]*. In a few moments I will ask you to open your eyes in order to watch the film. Stay as hypnotized as you are now, open your eyes and watch the film.' When video ends 'Please close your eyes now–and return to your special place.'

ii. Script for Suggested Dissociation Condition

Stay as hypnotized as you are now with your eyes closed–imagine that you are looking at a television screen–begin to have the experience of the screen in front of you. *[Pause. Participant is asked to signal with a head nod when this has been achieved]*. As you do that begin to have the experience of looking at the screen but of seeing it from a different perspective as though you are viewing it from outside your own body–from a different point of view–looking at the screen and being aware of yourself looking at the screen almost as though you were another person . . . being aware of the screen and being aware of yourself watching it. As you continue to look at the screen, everything around you beginning to seem strange and unreal as though you were somehow another person in a strange place. Begin to have that feeling of being outside yourself and of the screen and surroundings being unfamiliar *[Pause. Participant is asked to signal with a head nod when this has been achieved]*. Good just let those feelings of being outside yourself develop further as you watch the screen–and those feelings of the screen and your surroundings being unfamiliar and unreal becoming stronger and clearer–until they are as strong as they can be for you just now. *[Pause. Participant is asked to signal with a head nod when this has been achieved]*. In a few moments I will ask you to open your eyes in order to watch the film. When you open your eyes continue to have those feelings as you watch what is shown on the screen–being fully aware of the events taking place in the film–watching what happens as though you are viewing it from outside your own body. . . what is shown on the screen feeling strange and unreal as though you were someone else watching what is happening–all the time paying full attention to what is being shown on the screen whilst watching it from another perspective . . . Continue to have these feelings for the whole time you watch the film until you are given different instructions. Stay as hypnotized as you are now, open your eyes and watch the film.

When video ends 'Please close your eyes now–returning to normal feelings, experiencing the world from your own perspective–everything feeling as real and normal as it should *[Pause. Participant is asked to signal with a head nod when this has been achieved]*. Return now to your special place.'

Dissociation: Cognitive Capacity or Dysfunction?

Michiel B. de Ruiter, PhD
Bernet M. Elzinga, PhD
R. Hans Phaf, PhD

SUMMARY. Dissociative experiences are mostly studied as a risk factor for dissociative pathology. Nonpathological dissociation is quite common in the general population, however, and may reflect a constitutionally determined cognitive style rather than a pathological trait acquired through the experience of adverse life events. In a theoretical model, we propose that nonpathological dissociation is characterized by high levels of elaboration learning and reconstructive retrieval, for which enhanced levels of attentional and working memory abilities are a prerequisite. These characteristics, in general, seem to be representative for a higher ability to (re-)construct conscious experiences. We review

Michiel B. de Ruiter is affiliated with the Psychiatry Department, Academic Medical Center, Amsterdam, The Netherlands, and the VU University, Department of Clinical Neuropsychology, Amsterdam, The Netherlands.

Bernet M. Elzinga is affiliated with the Section of Clinical and Health Psychology, University of Leiden, The Netherlands.

R. Hans Phaf is affiliated with the Department of Psychonomics, University of Amsterdam, Amsterdam, The Netherlands.

Address correspondence to: Michiel B. de Ruiter, Department of Clinical Neuropsychology, VU University, Van der Boechorststraat 1, 1081 BT Amsterdam, The Netherlands (E-mail: mb.de.ruiter@psy.vu.nl).

[Haworth co-indexing entry note]: "Dissociation: Cognitive Capacity or Dysfunction?" de Ruiter, Michiel B., Bernet M. Elzinga, and R. Hans Phaf. Co-published simultaneously in *Journal of Trauma & Dissociation* (The Haworth Medical Press, an imprint of The Haworth Press, Inc.) Vol. 7, No. 4, 2006, pp. 115-134; and: *Exploring Dissociation: Definitions, Development and Cognitive Correlates* (ed: Anne P. DePrince, and Lisa DeMarni Cromer) The Haworth Medical Press, an imprint of The Haworth Press, Inc., 2006, pp. 115-134. Single or multiple copies of this article are available for a fee from The Haworth Document Delivery Service [1-800-HAWORTH, 9:00 a.m. - 5:00 p.m. (EST). E-mail address: docdelivery@haworthpress.com].

some of our behavioral as well as neural (i.e., fMRI, ERPs) studies, suggesting that high dissociative individuals are characterized by heightened levels of attention, working memory and episodic memory. In nonpathological conditions a person may benefit from these dissociative abilities, although after adverse (e.g., traumatic) events the disposition may develop into dissociative pathology. doi:10.1300/J229v07n04_07 *[Article copies available for a fee from The Haworth Document Delivery Service: 1-800-HAWORTH. E-mail address: <docdelivery@haworthpress.com> Website: <http://www.HaworthPress.com> © 2006 by The Haworth Press, Inc. All rights reserved.]*

KEYWORDS. Dissociation, elaboration, construction, working memory, attention, episodic memory

    Dissociation can be broadly defined as a structured separation of mental processes that are ordinarily integrated (Spiegel & Cardeña, 1991). The term is best known as the pathological coping mechanism by which some psychiatric patients 'block' (i.e., dissociate) traumatic memories from entering conscious awareness, a condition known as dissociative amnesia. The veracity of these 'lost memories' has been the subject of a grim debate known as the 'memory wars' (Schacter, 1995). In contrast to this rare and controversial pathological phenomenon, it has often been suggested that dissociative experiences are common in everyday life (Kihlstrom, Glisky, & Angiulo, 1994; Ray, 1996), and may relate to certain characteristics of nonpathological information processing. A person may, for instance, be so engaged in watching a movie, that she does not notice another person entering the room. Apparently, the current surroundings are–temporarily–dissociated from awareness. This benign form of dissociation is sometimes called absorption. Epidemiological studies report that dissociative experiences as measured with dissociation questionnaires (e.g., DES, Bernstein & Putnam, 1986, Dis-Q, Vanderlinden, Van Dyck, Vandereycken, Vertommen, & Verkes, 1993) are quite common in the general population (e.g., Putnam et al., 1996; Ross, Joshi, & Currie, 1990; Vanderlinden, Van Dyck, Vandereycken, & Vertommen, 1991). Moreover, twin studies have identified a strong genetic component in dissociation (Becker-Blease, Deater-Deckard, Eley, Freyd, Stevenson, & Plomin, 2004; Jang, Paris, Zweig-Frank, & Livesley, 1998), which suggests that dissociative experiences may occur, at least to some extent, independently from adverse life events.

    It has been argued that nonpathological dissociative tendencies might in some circumstances (i.e., traumatic experiences) constitute a risk factor for developing pathological dissociation (Kihlstrom et al., 1994). Several studies have reported a relation between childhood abuse and adult dissociation (Chu & Dill, 1990; Mulder, Beautrais, Joyce, & Fergusson, 1998). When faced, therefore, with stressful situations, basic cognitive characteristics of high-dissociative, healthy individuals may become a risk factor that predisposes for developing dissociative psychopathology.

In spite of its pathological connotation, in *non*clinical subjects dissociation may primarily constitute a cognitive trait which varies naturally in the population and is not necessarily associated with the experience of trauma. According to our view, nonpathological dissociation reflects an important general information processing style, associated with enhanced attention and working memory capacities. In the following, we will first describe the theoretical background of the *construction hypothesis* on dissociation, which postulates that high dissociators are better at constructing conscious experiences due to enhanced elaboration learning, for which attention and working memory are prerequisites. We then present a short overview of the empirical studies on attention and memory functioning in nonclinical and clinical subjects, followed by a summary of the empirical studies from our group that directly investigated this theoretical model.

DISSOCIATION, ELABORATION LEARNING AND (RE)CONSTRUCTION

In several previous writings, dissociation has already been mentioned in relation to basic attentional and working memory abilities. Braun and Sachs (1985), for example, in their book chapter on predisposing factors for the development of what was then called Multiple Personality Disorder (now relabeled as Dissociative Identity Disorder in the DSM-IV), already suggested that a "natural, inborn capacity to dissociate" (p. 42) characterized individuals that had developed this disorder later on in life, and that this ability operated in relation with several additional features including an "excellent working memory" (p. 44). The observation, moreover, that dissociation is related to "the capacity to ignore extrinsic stimuli" (Jang et al., 1998) clearly suggests that basic attentional abilities are an important component of dissociation.

In line with these earlier observations, we propose that high-dissociative nonclinical individuals are characterized by heightened levels of elaborative processing of information or memories, leading to heightened levels of conscious memory (see Elzinga et al., 2000). These ideas are based on the activation/elaboration theories from Mandler (1980; 1985; 2002). According to Mandler, activation learning is the strengthening of existing associations and mainly contributes to non-conscious memory performance. Elaboration learning, on the other hand, consists in the formation of new associations and forms a prerequisite for conscious memory performance. Elaboration may take place during both encoding and retrieval, and can best be characterized as a constructive memory process. As conscious recollection is per definition a reconstruction of events, it need not be an exact reproduction, as if some video report has been made. A higher tendency to elaboratively encode and reconstruct ('retrieve') information or experiences may lead to a higher conscious memory performance, but may at the same time be associated with an enhanced sensitivity for 'false positives,' i.e., memory constructions that include new associations that were not present in the original situation, as in false memories. False recollection seems to mirror veridical recollection in this respect. Deeper levels of encoding, for instance, increase both types of recollection (e.g., Thapar & McDermott, 2001). Similarly, we propose that dissociative tendencies enhance both veridical and false recollection. Furthermore, it is proposed that constructive processes will emerge most clearly while processing 'concern relevant' information, being either challenging or complex, or information that is related to personal goals, fears, or adverse events.

As mentioned earlier, the two basic cognitive skills that seem to lie at the heart of dissociative abilities are attention and working memory. Many theorists have postulated strong bidirectional links between attention and working memory (e.g., Awh & Jonides, 2001; De Fockert, Rees, Frith, & Lavie, 2001; Downing, 2000; Kane & Engle, 2003). Conway, Cowan, and Bunting (2001), for instance, have suggested that a low working memory span corresponds to impaired inhibition of distracting information in attentional tasks. Conversely, words that are kept active longer in working memory are generally encoded more strongly in episodic memory (e.g., Raaijmakers & Shiffrin, 1981). Because attentional and working memory skills are a prerequisite for elaborative encoding, high dissociators should in our view, be characterized by a large working memory span and high attentional abilities. More specifically, we propose that high dissociators are characterized by heightened levels of attention and working memory capacity, resulting in higher levels of elaboration and reconstruction. Below, we will review existing studies on attention and memory on dissociation, and then report studies conducted by our group that have specifically tested the construction hypothesis.

STUDIES ON ATTENTION AND DISSOCIATION

Relatively few studies have directly investigated the role of attention related to dissociation. In one of the first studies investigating a sample of college students, Freyd, Martorello, Avarado, Hayes, and Christman (1998) found that high dissociators were characterized by more classical Stroop interference than low dissociators. Extending their paradigm with a divided attention condition, in which participants were instructed to name the color of the presented words and at the same time try to remember them, DePrince and Freyd (1999) found that high dissociators tended to show more Stroop interference in the selective attention condition and less interference in the divided attention condition, suggesting enhanced attentional capacities in the divided attention situation. DePrince and Freyd argued that a dual task information processing style may develop as a consequence of trauma (typically sexual abuse in childhood by a caregiver). This dissociative style would be apparent in daily life situations that are not related to the experienced trauma.

Another line of research used the Flanker paradigm to investigate negative priming in DID and other patient groups (Dorahy, Irwin, & Middleton, 2002; Dorahy, Irwin, & Middleton, 2004; Dorahy, McCusker, Loewenstein, Colbert, & Mulholland, 2006; Dorahy, Middleton, & Irwin, 2004; Dorahy, Middleton, & Irwin, 2005). In most of their experiments, participants were instructed to name centrally presented numbers and ignore peripherally presented numbers (e.g., '2 3 2' was presented and '3' had to be named). On a consecutive trial, a different set of numbers was presented (e.g., '9 5 9') or a set of numbers was presented with the central stimulus being the number that had to be ignored previously (e.g., '1 2 1'). The increase in reaction time that usually occurs during the latter trial type is called negative priming and is taken as an index of the capacity to ignore irrelevant stimuli, and thus, of selective attention (although it should be noted that Dorahy and colleagues discuss their results in terms of working memory functioning). DID patients generally showed high levels of negative priming (sometimes numerically higher than normal control groups: Dorahy, Irwin, & Middleton, 2004; Dorahy et al., 2005; Dorahy et al., 2006), indicating a high level of cognitive inhibition. These effects disappeared, however, when the flanker stimuli were intermixed with affectively negative words (Dorahy et al., 2005; Dorahy et al., 2006). Dorahy interpreted these effects as evidence that cognitive inhibitory processes of selective attention covary in dissociation with the level of state anxiety experienced, i.e., weakened inhibition in anxiety-provoking situations. They suggested that with reduced inhibition, more streams of information can be given more intense processing.

STUDIES ON DECLARATIVE MEMORY AND DISSOCIATION

A number of studies has been conducted on memory functioning in traumatized individuals with varying levels of dissociative symptoms, including college students (DePrince and Freyd, 2001, 2004), patients with Dissociative Identity Disorder (Elzinga, de Beurs, Sergeant, Van Dyck, & Phaf, 2000; Elzinga, Phaf, Ardon, & Van Dyck, 2003), PTSD (McNally, Metzger, Lasko, Clancy, & Pitman, 1998), Acute Stress Disorder (Moulds & Bryant, 2002, 2005), Borderline Personality Disorder (Cloitre, Cancienne, Brodsky, Dulit, & Perry,1996; Korfine & Hooley, 2000), and women with continuous or recovered memories of childhood sexual abuse (McNally, Clancy, & Schacter, 2001; McNally, Ristuccia, & Perlman, 2005). These studies aimed to examine mechanisms underlying psychogenic amnesia for traumatic experiences using the 'directed forgetting' paradigm. In this paradigm, participants are cued to remember or forget trauma-related and control words (i.e., generally emotional and affectively neutral), hypothesizing that individuals with psychogenic amnesia are better at forgetting trauma-related information (see Cloitre, 1992). In general, it has proven hard to find indications of memory impairment for trauma-related stimuli in high-dissociative individuals with a reported history of childhood abuse (e.g., McNally et al., 1998; 2001; 2005), adding little support to the idea that they are characterized by an avoidant encoding strategy (Cloitre, 1992). In contrast, the only study involving DID-patients found that DID-patients (when tested within the same 'state') showed higher levels of recollection (for emotional, sex-related words) compared to controls (Elzinga et al., 2000), which was also found among BPD patients with high dissociative symptomatology (Cloitre et al., 1996; Korfine & Hooley, 2000). The studies that did find directed forgetting of trauma words are in patients with Acute Stress Disorder (Moulds & Bryant, 2002, 2005) and in high-dissociative college students, in which enhanced forgetting of trauma words was found under divided attention conditions (DePrince and Freyd, 2001, 2005). A study among women with recovered and continuous memories of childhood sexual abuse could not replicate the enhanced forgetting of trauma words under divided attention conditions, however (McNally et al., 2005).

Higher levels of conscious recollection in individuals with a high-dissociative personality trait should be contrasted to the general impairments in explicit memory (but not implicit memory) in patients with dissociative identity disorder when memory functioning is tested after changing personality state (Eich, Macauley, Loewenstein, & Dihle, 1997; Elzinga et al., 2003, but see Huntjens, Postma, Peters, Woertman, van der Hart, 2003). More pertinent to the present issue, however, Silberman, Putnam, Weingartner, Braun, and Post (1985) found that together with impaired free recall and recognition in a dissociative condition (i.e., after a change of 'alter') relative to healthy controls mimicking a dissociative state change dissociative patients showed again a much higher level of memory performance than controls in the non-dissociative condition (i.e., without state change). Still, it should be noted that the experimental procedures were not equal for patients and controls, i.e., patients heard stimuli twice in the nondissociative condition. Therefore, these results should be interpreted with caution.

Taken together, one might conclude that dissociation is not related to enhanced forgetting of trauma-related information using the directed forgetting paradigm, and might even be related to enhanced recall, as in the case of DID patients. In most studies, it is impossible, however, to disentangle to role of psychiatric status and trauma history from the role of trait dissociation on memory functioning. As trauma history combined with psychiatric status is likely to have detrimental effects on memory performance (e.g., because of concentration problems and/or neurological damage) and cognitive functioning in general, one could suspect that this may have disguised the effects of increased elaboration related to dissociation. Moreover, patient groups are often older and have lower educational levels, two characteristics that are also likely to have detrimental effects on memory performance.

STUDIES ON MEMORY INTRUSIONS AND DISSOCIATION

Another line of research related to memory and dissociation originates from the debate on the veracity of recovered memories (Schacter, 1995), initiating studies that investigated whether high-dissociative individuals might be more prone to develop 'false' memories than low-dissociative individuals. In several studies, a higher liability to report false childhood memories has been found in nonclinical high dissociative individuals (Hyman & Billings, 1998; Ost, Foster, Costall, & Bull, 2005). A similar positive relation has, moreover, been reported using a misinformation paradigm (Cann & Katz, 2005). The classic Deese-Roediger-McDermott (DRM) or 'critical lure' paradigm has also been used to study illusory memories in the laboratory (e.g., Roediger & McDermott, 2000). In the critical lure paradigm, semantically related words are presented at study, after which the words are intermixed with semantically associated items that have not been presented before ('lures'). It was found that high levels of dissociative experiences were related to increased recall of neutral critical lures being erroneously identified as previously presented in the list in women with reported sexual abuse and PTSD (Bremner, Shobe, & Kihlstrom, 2000), and in women reporting recovered memories of sexual abuse (but no PTSD), (Clancy, Schacter, McNally, & Pitman, 2000). More recently, evidence was also reported for enhanced recall of critical lures of trauma-related words in women reporting recovered memories of childhood sexual abuse (Geraerts, Smeets, Jelicic, van Heerden, & Merckelbach, 2005).

With respect to illusory memory studies including the DRM effect, no studies have reported a reduction in recollection of critical lures for high dissociators, while most studies have shown a positive relation with these constructs. This fits with findings that in several studies, positive correlations have been reported between dissociation and fantasy proneness and related constructs (Merckelbach, Muris, Horselenberg, & Stougie, 2000; Merckelbach, Horselenberg, & Schmidt, 2002; Elzinga, Bermondt, & Van Dyck, 2002). Taken together, these findings are consistent with the view that a heightened elaborative encoding and retrieval ability in high dissociators is responsible for both increased veridical and illusory recollection.

EMPIRICAL STUDIES ON THE CONSTRUCTION HYPOTHESIS

In a series of experiments, we aimed to directly investigate the construction hypothesis on dissociation, measuring basic information processing characteristics of dissociative tendencies in the normal population. To this end, college students were selected that scored in the high vs. low ranges on a dissociation questionnaire (Dis-Q; Vanderlinden et al., 1993). These participants performed several tasks on attention, working memory and declarative memory. Our general hypothesis was that dissociative tendencies in healthy individuals are not related to aberrant cognitive functioning or to traumatic experiences, but instead reflect a distinct information processing style that, in general, is related to enhanced memory and attention functions.

Dissociation and Working Memory

Firstly, verbal working memory span was examined for affectively neutral words, using a Dutch version of the word span test of Daneman and Carpenter (1980) in a large sample of low, medium and high-dissociative nonclinical psychology students (De Ruiter, Phaf, Elzinga, & Van Dyck, 2004). This test was composed of sets of short familiar words that were as semantically and phonetically unrelated as possible. Sets of increasing size were read out by the experimenter and the participant had to recall these words aloud in the exact order of presentation. The largest set of words that could be recalled this way was taken as a measure for working memory span. As expected, we found that the verbal span of the high-dissociative group was significantly larger than of the medium- and low-dissociative groups.

To further investigate the role of working memory in dissociative subjects, we studied the role of maintenance and manipulation of working memory related to dissociation, and investigated the brain areas involved. To this end, two working memory tasks (the Sternberg task and the N-back task) were presented to low and high dissociators while measuring functional Magnetic Resonance Images (fMRI; Veltman et al., 2005). In the Sternberg task, participants were instructed to memorize a letter string of varying length (2-7 letters) after which the string disappeared and single letters were projected on a screen. Participants were requested to indicate with a key press whether the letter had been in the string. In the N-back task, participants saw single letters projected on a screen and were requested to press a key when the projected letter was an 'X' (baseline condition), the same as the last shown (1-back), the same as the letter preceding the last shown (2-back) or the same as the letter preceding the last two shown (3-back). To prevent fatigue, the N-back task consisted of two subsessions. Behavioral data demonstrated that high-dissociators performed better during the Sternberg task as well as during the second sub-session of the N-back task. In addition, for both tasks, more task-load related increase in activity in the left dorsolateral prefrontal cortex (DLPFC) was found for high than low dissociators (see Figure 1 for a visualization of fMRI activity during the

FIGURE 1. Three-dimensional rendering of task-load-related fMRI activity during the Sternberg task for low dissociators (left panel) and high dissociators (right panel). L = left hemisphere, R = right hemisphere. Reprinted from Veltman, D. J., de Ruiter, M. B., Rombouts, S. A. R. B., Lazeron, R. H. C., Barkhof, F., Van Dyck, R., Dolan, R. J., & Phaf, R. H. (2005). Neurophysiological correlates of increased verbal working memory in high-dissociative participants: A functional MRI study. *Psychological Medicine*, 35(02), pp. 175-185, with permission from Cambridge University Press.

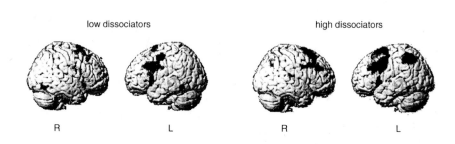

Sternberg task). Because this brain structure is consistently activated in working memory tasks, these results suggest that high-dissociative participants recruit brain areas responsible for working memory functioning to a greater extent, which was associated with better task performance.

Taken together, we found behavioral evidence that high dissociators are characterized by a higher working memory capacity as indexed by three different types of working memory tasks. These behavioral results were corroborated by fMRI data showing more task load-related increase in activity in dorsolateral prefrontal cortex for high than low dissociators. Interestingly, in a recent study, Elzinga, Ardon, Heijnis, de Ruiter, van Dyck, and Veltman (submitted) replicated these effects in a group of patients with dissociative disorders, finding enhanced activation in the DLPFC for dissociative patients and a relative lower increase in number of errors with increasing task load compared to healthy controls. This suggests that a high working memory span is also characteristic for individuals suffering from pathological dissociation. This is remarkable given the fact that these patients were highly stressed and anxious, which outside the context of dissociation, has been found to have detrimental effects on verbal working memory (Klein & Boals, 2001; Elzinga & Roelofs, 2005; Gray, 2001). Our results apparently contradict the conjecture by Dorahy et al. (2006), who proposed that patients with dissociative disorders suffer from working memory deficits in high-anxiety situations.

DISSOCIATION AND ATTENTION

To examine the influence of dissociative tendencies on the time course of attentional processes, EEG-derived Event-Related Potentials (ERPs) were measured in the encoding phase of a deep/shallow encoding paradigm (De Ruiter, Phaf, Veltman, Kok, & Van Dyck, 2003). Presenting affectively negative and neutral words, participants had to give a valence judgment (deep encoding) or detect the letter 'A' (shallow encoding) in the presented words. The deep/shallow paradigm may provide a more ecologically valid approach to measure dissociative abilities compared to the directed forgetting studies. In directed forgetting studies, participants are instructed to either remember or forget a stimulus *after* it has appeared on the screen, whereas in the deep/shallow encoding paradigm, the attention of the participant is directed to or away from the meaning of the stimulus *during* stimulus presentation. Moreover, this paradigm constitutes an incidental learning paradigm (as opposed to an intentional paradigm in directed forgetting studies), which has the additional advantage that participants are not aware their memory will be tested later on in the experimental session.

When high-dissociative participants had to detect the letter 'A,' enhanced ERP amplitudes and short reaction times indicated that high dissociators were characterized by enhanced focusing of attention to this stimulus feature compared to low dissociators. The fact that these effects were also present for affectively neutral words indicates that this heightened attention in high dissociators was independent of affective processing: neither the stimulus, neither the task at hand (letter detection) seem to be emotion-dependent. Moreover, a negative affective stimulus valence did have an effect on high dissociators in the attentional task: in high dissociators the detection of the letter A was faster, and the concomitant ERP component larger for negatively than neutrally valenced words, indicating increased focusing of attention to this stimulus category. This effect was not observed in low dissociators (see Figure 2). This effect may be due to the intrinsic attention capturing properties of emotional words compared to neutral words, inducing more elaboration in the high dissociators.

FIGURE 2. Grand average ERP waveforms at Pz (electrode located at middle parietal cortex) for low dissociators (left panel) and high dissociators (right panel) during the letter detection task. Depicted are ERPs to neutral words containing the letter A, neutral words not containing the letter A, negative words containing the letter A, and negative words not containing the letter A. Reprinted from De Ruiter, M. B., Phaf, R. H., Veltman, D. J., Kok, A., & Van Dyck, R. (2003). Attention as a characteristic of nonclinical dissociation: an event-related potential study. *Neuroimage, 19,* 376-390, with permission from Elsevier.

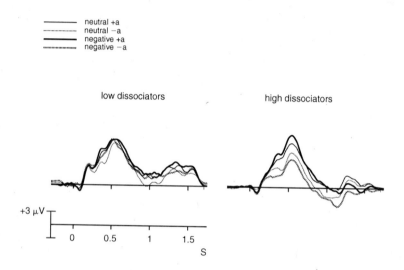

Probably as a result of their high working memory capacity, high dissociators were able to perform the primary task and at the same time pay attention to the affective valence of the stimuli, indicating a superior ability to divide attention as well. Alternatively, the effect might be due to a higher anxiety of the high dissociators (we did not obtain anxiety measures in this study). However, we find it more probable that anxiety would have *interfering* effects on stimulus encoding, which would be apparent as a increase instead of decrease of reaction times. A recent study from our group (Phaf, Stienen, & de Ruiter, submitted) on the role of dissociation in implicit memory processes suggests that enhanced attention may not be specifically related to negative information. In an exclusion task (c.f., Merikle, Joordens & Stolz, 1995), words were presented for variable durations that were sometimes very short (in our study, the durations were 29, 43, 57, 71 and 214 ms). Subsequently, a word stem was presented and participants were asked to complete the word stem with another word than the one that had been presented (i.e., to exclude the previously seen word from completion). For instance, the word 'pancake' was presented for the very short duration of 43 ms, and then, 'pan' was shown on the screen. If the participant completed this stem with 'cake,' this was taken as an indication that unconscious memory processes were involved: the participant had no conscious experience of the word 'pancake' (otherwise she would have excluded the word), but pancake was the first word that came to mind. If, on the other hand, the participant completed this stem with another word (e.g., 'panther'), this was taken as an indication that conscious memory was involved: the participant consciously perceived the word 'pancake' and therefore knew she has to come up with another word that starts with 'pan.' In this paradigm, word stems were also presented without a word preceding it (e.g., 'pan' was presented without 'pancake' preceding it). Completion levels for words on these trials were taken as a measure for baseline performance with which performance on the other trials was compared. We found that both exclusion failure (i.e., above-baseline completion at short durations) and exclusion success (i.e., below-baseline completion at longer durations) were shifted to shorter durations for high-dissociative nonclinical participants, equally with positive, neutral, and negative words. Dissociative ability, thus, appears to facilitate perception and identification of all kinds of words, irrespective of word valence.

DISSOCIATION AND RECOLLECTION

Because ERPs provide information about the time course of neural processing in a millisecond resolution, they are perfectly suited to index early occurring and fast changing processes like attention. On the other hand, fMRI is the designated measure to indicate where in the brain cognitive functions are located. In a deep encoding task, where participants had to judge the affective valence of neutral and negative words, fMRI data indicated an increase of activation in ventrolateral prefrontal cortex (one of the locations where working memory is thought to reside) and the hippocampus (a pivotal structure in intermediate memory storage and memory retrieval) in response to negatively valenced words, with this effect being stronger for high than low dissociators (De Ruiter, 2005; De Ruiter, Veltman, Phaf, & Van Dyck, submitted). It thus seems that elaborative encoding of negatively valenced stimuli was stronger for high than low dissociators. Corroborating the encoding results, in the recognition task, we found that high dissociators showed better memory performance (i.e., sensitivity) for negatively valence words than low dissociators. Moreover, group differences in favor of the high dissociators in the left and right posterior hippocampus and the inferior parietal lobule complex were found during retrieval. Next to the hippocampus, the inferior parietal lobule complex is also associated with conscious recollection (e.g., Shannon & Buckner, 2004). These effects did not depend on affective stimulus valence. Therefore, these data suggest that high dissociators are characterized by high levels of conscious recollection.

CONCLUSION:
DISSOCIATION: COGNITIVE CAPACITY OR DYSFUNCTION?

Dissociative style in nonclinical subjects appears to be a powerful individual difference, in the sense that it corresponds to a number of differences in information processing in a variety of experimental paradigms, including attention, working memory and episodic memory. As reviewed, dissociation has been found to be related to both enhanced veridical and enhanced false memories. One of the questions that may arise is therefore whether dissociative tendencies are best considered as a capacity or a dysfunction. The answer to the question seems to be a matter of taste. In any case, the observed relations between dissociation, memory illusions, fantasy proneness, and absent-mindedness are not in disagreement with our findings of high attentional and working memory abilities. Apparently, the benefits of constructive capacities may be accompanied by the costs of cognitive failures, such as incorrect memory constructions. Still, it is easy to conceive that mental processes like absent-mindedness and fantasy proneness may be detrimental for task performance: if somebody is not paying attention to a particular task, she is not going to perform well on this task. Illustrative in this respect is a study by Giesbrecht, Merckelbach, Geraerts, and Smeets (2004), in which participants differing in their scores on the DES were asked to perform a Random Number Generation task in which they had to generate random sequences of numbers ranging from 1 to 10. Modest positive correlations (in the range of 0.2) were found between scores on two subscales of the DES (DES-T and amnesia) and certain patterns that were held to be deviations from randomness, e.g., repeating of the same number. An important issue at stake here seems to be motivation: if the task is sufficiently demanding high dissociators may display superior performance on basic attention and memory paradigms. If not, high dissociators may easily divert their high working memory capacity to more interesting (mental) activities like daydreaming. This is in line with the finding that in some working memory tasks (Veltman et al., 2005), superior performance of the high dissociators became apparent only for higher task loads. The same holds for the finding of DePrince & Freyd (1999) that high dissociators perform better under the more challenging divided attention conditions. On the other hand, the letter detection task (detecting the letter 'A') was fairly easy to accomplish, and high dissociators also displayed improved performance on this task compared to low dissociators. The letter detection task, however, was relatively short and subjective reports from participants indicated that the task was quite entertaining to perform. Taken together, one might conclude that nonclinical dissociation may be related to enhanced attentional and memory capacities, provided that the task is complex or challenging enough to capture the attention.

Second, the view that nonpathological dissociative ability may reflect a largely inborn capacity contrasts in some respects with the idea that a dissociative coping style may develop as a consequence of trauma (typically sexual abuse in childhood by a caregiver), which eventually may lead to a dual task information processing style (De Prince & Freyd, 1999). This dissociative style would be apparent in daily life situations not necessarily related to the experienced trauma. In this view, performance differences between nonclinical low and high dissociators on basic attention tasks are primarily the result of differences in trauma history. In favor of the idea that dissociative differences may occur, at least to some extent, independently from adverse life events, it can be mentioned that twin studies have identified a strong genetic component in dissociation (Becker-Blease et al., 2004; Jang et al., 1998). Moreover, with regard to the data reported here, it seems unlikely that the behavioral and neural characteristics of high-dissociative college students are primarily related to trauma history. Firstly, it is improbable that trauma history would result in superior performance across a wide range of basic cognitive tasks that are, for the most part, not related to affective stimulus material or affective processing. Moreover, in traumatized individuals many memory functions, including working memory and declarative memory for neutral information is impaired (Elzinga & Bremner, 2002). In our view, it is more likely that high dissociative nonclinical individuals elaborate more on information that attracts their attention, be it emotionally negative or positive material (as in the shallow/deep encoding task or exclusion task), or complex material (as in the working memory tasks).

It may be very likely, however, particularly when emotional experiences are involved, that eminent dissociative abilities may be invoked to cope with the urgent and personally relevant circumstances that are usually associated with emotions, and that exposure to severe or chronic traumatic experience, may increases this dissociative ability. Individuals with high dissociative abilities might be prone to develop dissociative disorders when exposed to traumatic events, whereas individuals without dissociative tendencies might develop depressive symptoms, PTSD, borderline personality or psychotic features. Tragically, dissociative patients may also be more liable to higher levels of false recollections, which may damage their credibility. Nonpathological individuals with high dissociative tendencies may, however, profit from their abilities, for instance by a higher level of intelligence (i.e., working memory performance forms a part of most intelligence tests, Ackerman, Beier, & Boyle, 2005). In general, it seems that dissociation should not in the first place be considered a characteristic of a disorder, but might rather be seen as a distinct ability that may be beneficial in many conditions.

REFERENCES

Ackerman, P. L., Beier, M. E., & Boyle, M. O. (2005). Working memory and intelligence: the same or different constructs? *Psychological Bulletin, 131*, 30-60.

Awh, E., & Jonides, J. (2001). Overlapping mechanisms of attention and spatial working memory. *Trends in Cognitive Sciences, 5*, 119-126.

Becker-Blease, K. A., Deater-Deckard, K., Eley, T., Freyd, J. F., Stevenson, J., & Plomin, R. (2004). A genetic analysis of individual differences in dissociative behaviours in childhood and adolescence. *Journal of Child Psychology and Psychiatry, 45*, 522-532.

Bernstein, E. M., & Putnam, F. W. (1986). Development, reliability, and validity of a dissociation scale. *Journal of Nervous and Mental Disease, 174*, 727-735.

Braun, B. G., & Sachs, R. G. (1985). The development of multiple personality disorder: Predisposing, precipitating, and perpetuating factors. In: Kluft, R. P. (Ed.), *Childhood antecedents of multiple personality disorder*. American Psychiatric Press, Washington, DC, pp. 37-64.

Bremner, J. D., Shobe, K. K., & Kihlstrom, J. F. (2000). False memories in women with self-reported childhood sexual abuse: An empirical study. *Psychological Science, 11*, 333-337.

Cann, D. R., & Katz, A. N. (2005). Habitual acceptance of misinformation: Examination of individual differences and source attributions. *Memory & Cognition, 33,* 405-417.

Chu, J. A., & Dill, D. L. (1990). Dissociative symptoms in relation to childhood physical and sexual abuse. *American Journal of Psychiatry, 147,* 887-892.

Clancy, S., Schacter, D., McNally, R., & Pitman, R. K. (2000). False recognition in women reporting recovered memories of sexual abuse. *Psychological Science, 11,* 26-31.

Cloitre, M. (1992). Avoidance of emotional processing: A cognitive perspective. In D. J. Stein & J. E. Young (Eds.), *Cognitive science and clinical disorders* (pp. 19-41). San Diego, CA: Academic Press.

Cloitre, M., Cancienne, J., Brodsky, B., Dulit, R., & Perry, S. W. (1996). Memory performance among women with parental abuse histories: Enhanced directed forgetting or directed remembering? *Journal of Abnormal Psychology, 105,* 204-211.

Conway, A. R. A., Cowan, N., & Bunting, M. F. (2001). The cocktail party phenomenon revisited: The importance of working memory capacity. *Psychonomic Bulletin and Review, 8,* 331-335.

Daneman, M., & Carpenter, P. A. (1980). Individual differences in working memory and reading. *Journal of Verbal Learning and Verbal Behavior, 19,* 450-466.

De Fockert, J. W., Rees, G., Frith, C. D., & Lavie, N. (2001). The role of working memory in visual selective attention. *Science, 291,* 1803-1806.

De Ruiter, M. B. (2005). Neural correlates of nonclinical dissociation. Unpublished doctoral dissertation, University of Amsterdam, The Netherlands.

De Ruiter, M. B., Phaf, R. H., Elzinga, B. M., & Van Dyck, R. (2004). Dissociative style and individual differences in verbal working memory span. *Consciousness and Cognition, 13,* 821-828.

De Ruiter, M. B., Phaf, R. H., Veltman, D. J., Kok, A., & Van Dyck, R. (2003). Attention as a characteristic of nonclinical dissociation: An event-related potential study. *Neuroimage, 19,* 376-390.

De Ruiter, M. B., Veltman, D. J., Phaf, R. H., & Van Dyck, R. (submitted). Negative words enhance recognition in nonclinical high dissociators: An fMRI study.

DePrince, A. P., & Freyd, J. J. (1999). Dissociative tendencies, attention, and memory. *Psychological Science, 10,* 449-452.

DePrince, A. P. & Freyd, J. J. (2001). Memory and dissociative tendencies: The roles of attentional context and word meaning in a directed forgetting task. *Journal of Trauma & Dissociation, 2,* 67-82.

DePrince, A. P., & Freyd, J. J. (2004). Forgetting trauma stimuli. *Psychological Science, 15,* 488-492.

D'Esposito, M., Detre, J. A., Alsop, D. C., Shin, R. K., Atlas, S., & Grossman, M. (1995). The neural basis of the central executive system of working memory. *Nature, 378,* 279-281.

Dorahy, M. J., Irwin, H. J., & Middleton, W. (2002). Cognitive inhibition in dissociative identity disorder (DID): Developing an understanding of working memory function in DID. *Journal of Trauma and Dissociation, 3,* 111-132.

Dorahy, M. J., Irwin, H. J., & Middleton, W. (2004). Assessing markers of working memory function in dissociative identity disorder using neutral stimuli: A comparison with clinical and general population samples. *Australian and New Zealand Journal of Psychiatry, 38,* 47-55.

Dorahy, M. J., McCuskerb, C. G., Loewenstein, R. J., Colbert, K., & Mulholland, C. (2006). Cognitive inhibition and interference in dissociative identity disorder: The effects of anxiety on specific executive functions. *Behaviour Research and Therapy, 44,* 749-764.

Dorahy, M. J., Middleton, W., & Irwin, H. J. (2004). Investigating cognitive inhibition in dissociative identity disorder compared to depression, posttraumatic stress disorder and schizophrenia. *Journal of Trauma and Dissociation, 5,* 93-110.

Dorahy, M. J., Middleton, W., & Irwin, H. J. (2005). The effect of emotional context on cognitive inhibition and attentional processing in dissociative identity disorder. *Behaviour Research and Therapy, 43,* 555-568.

Downing, P. E. (2000). Interactions between visual working memory and selective attention. *Psychological Science, 11,* 467-473.

Eich, E., Macauley, D., Loewenstein, R. J., & Dihle, P. H. (1997). Memory, amnesia and Dissociative Identity Disorder. *Psychological Science, 8,* 417-422.

Elzinga, B. M., Ardon, A. M., Heijnis, M. K., de Ruiter, M. B. van Dyck, R., & Veltman, D. J. (submitted). *Neural correlates of enhanced working memory performance in dissociative disorder: a functional MRI study.*

Elzinga, B. M., Bakker, A., Bremner, J. D. (2005). Stress-induced cortisol elevations are associated with impaired delayed, but not immediate recall. *Psychiatry Research, 30,* 211-223.

Elzinga, B. M., Bermond, B., & van Dyck, R. (2002). The relationship between dissociative proneness and alexithymia. *Psychotherapy and Psychosomatics, 71,* 104-111.

Elzinga, B. M., de Beurs, E., Sergeant, J. A., Van Dyck, R., & Phaf, R. H. (2000). Dissociative Style and Directed Forgetting. *Cognitive Therapy and Research, 24,* 279-295.

Elzinga, B. M., & Bremner, J. D. (2002). Are the neural substrates of memory the final common pathway in posttraumatic stress disorder (PTSD)? *Journal of Affective Disorders, 70,* 1-17.

Elzinga, B. M., Phaf, R. H., Ardon, A. M., & Van Dyck, R. (2003). Directed forgetting between but not within dissociative personality states. *Journal of Abnormal Psychology, 112,* 237-243.

Elzinga, B. M., & Roelofs, K. (2005). Cortisol-induced impairments of working memory require acute sympathetic activation. *Behavioral Neuroscience, 119,* 98-103.

Freyd, J. J., Martorello, S. R., Alvarado, J. S., Hayes, A. E., & Christman, J. C. (1998). Cognitive environments and dissociative tendencies: Performance on the standard stroop task for high versus low dissociators. *Applied Cognitive Psychology, 12,* S91-S103.

Geraerts, E., Smeets, E., Jelicic, M., van Heerden, J., & Merckelbach, H. (2005). Fantasy proneness, but not self-reported trauma is related to DRM performance of women reporting recovered memories of childhood sexual abuse. *Consciousness and Cognition, 14,* 602-612.

Giesbrecht, T., Merckelbach, H., Geraerts, E., & Smeets, E. (2004). Dissociation in undergraduate students: Disruptions in executive functioning. *The Journal of Nervous and Mental Disease, 192,* 567-569.

Gray, J. R. (2001). Emotional modulation of cognitive control: Approach-withdrawal states double-dissociate spatial from verbal two-back task performance. *Journal of Experimental Psychology: General, 130*, 436-452.

Huntjens, R. J., Postma, A., Peters, M. L., Woertman, L., & van der Hart, O. (2003). Interidentity amnesia for neutral, episodic information in dissociative identity disorder. *Journal of Abnormal Psychology, 112*, 290-297.

Hyman, I. E., & Billings, F. J. (1998). Individual differences and the creation of false memories. *Memory, 6*, 1-20.

Jang, K. L., Paris, J., Zweig-Frank, H., & Livesley, W. J. (1998). Twin study of dissociative experience. *Journal of Nervous and Mental Disease, 186*, 345-351.

Kane, M. J., & Engle, R. W. (2003). Working memory capacity and the control of attention: The contributions of goal neglect, response competition, and task set to Stroop interference. *Journal of Experimental Psychology, General, 132*, 47-70.

Kihlstrom, J. F., Glisky, M. L., & Angiulo, M. J. (1994). Dissociative tendencies and dissociative disorders. *Journal of Abnormal Psychology, 103*, 117-124.

Klein, K., & Boals, A. (2001). The relationship of life event stress and working memory capacity. *Applied Cognitive Psychology, 15*, 565-579.

Korfine, L., & Hooley, J. M. (2000). Directed forgetting of emotional stimuli in borderline personality disorder. *Journal of Abnormal Psychology, 109*, 214-221.

Mandler, G. (1980). Recognizing: The judgement of previous occurrence. *Psychological Review, 87*, 252-271.

Mandler, G. (1985). Cognitive psychology: An essay in cognitive science. Hillsdale, NJ: Erlbaum.

Mandler, G. (2002). *Consciousness recovered.* Amsterdam: John Benjamins.

McNally, R. J., Clancy, S. A., & Schacter, D. L. (2001). Directed forgetting of trauma cues in adults reporting repressed or recovered memories of childhood sexual abuse. *Journal of Abnormal Psychology, 110*, 151-156.

McNally, R. J., Metzger, L. J., Lasko, N. B., Clancy, S. A., & Pitman, R. K. (1998). Directed forgetting of trauma cues in adult survivors of childhood sexual abuse with and without posttraumatic stress disorder. *Journal of Abnormal Psychology, 107*, 596-601.

McNally, R. J., Ristuccia, C. S., & Perlman, C. A. (2005). Forgetting of trauma cues in adults reporting continuous or recovered memories of childhood sexual abuse. *Psychological Science, 16*, 336-340.

Merckelbach, H., Horselenberg, R., & Schmidt, H. (2002). Modeling the connection between self-reported trauma and dissociation in a student sample. *Personality and Individual Differences, 32*, 695-705.

Merckelbach, H., Muris, P., Horselenberg, R., & Stougie, S. (2000). Dissociative experiences, response bias, and fantasy proneness in college students. *Personality and Individual Differences, 28*, 49-58.

Merikle, P. M., Joordens, S., & Stolz, J. A. (1995). Measuring the relative magnitude of unconscious influences. *Consciousness and Cognition, 4*, 422-439.

Moulds, M. L., & Bryant, R. A. (2002). Directed forgetting in acute stress disorder. *Journal of Abnormal Psychology, 111*, 175-179.

Moulds, M. L., & Bryant, R. A. (2005). An investigation of retrieval inhibition in Acute Stress Disorder. *Journal of Traumatic Stress, 18*, 233-236.

Mulder, R. T., Beautrais, A. L., Joyce, P. R., & Fergusson, D. M. (1998). Relationship between dissociation, childhood sexual abuse, childhood physical abuse, and mental illness in a general population sample. *American Journal of Psychiatry, 55,* 806-811.

Ost, J., Foster, S., Costall, A., & Bull, R. (2005). False reports of childhood events in appropriate interviews. *Memory, 13,* 700-710.

Phaf, R. H., Stienen, B. M. C., & de Ruiter, M. B. (submitted). Dissociative ability facilitates word perception and identification.

Putnam, F. W., Carlson, E. B., Ross, C. A., Anderson, G., Clark, P., Torem, M., Bowman, E. S., Coons, P., Chu, J.A., Dill, D. L., Loewenstein, R. J., & Braun, B. G. (1996). Patterns of dissociation in clinical and nonclinical samples. *Journal of Nervous and Mental Disease, 184,* 673-679.

Raaijmakers, J. G. W., & Shiffrin, R. M. (1981). Search of associative memory. *Psychological Review, 88,* 552-572.

Ray, W. J. (1996). Dissociation in normal populations. In L. K. Michelson & W. J. Ray (Eds.), *Handbook of Dissociation: Theoretical, Empirical, and Clinical Perspectives.* (pp. 51-67). New York: Plenum Press.

Roediger, H. L., & McDermott, K. B. (2000). Tricks of memory. *Current Directions in Psychological Science, 9,* 123-127.

Ross, C. A., Joshi, S., & Currie, R. (1990). Dissociative experiences in the general population. *American Journal of Psychiatry, 147,* 1547-1552.

Schacter, D. L. (1995). Memory wars. *Scientific American, 272,* 135-139.

Shannon, B. J., Buckner, R. L. (2004). Functional-anatomic correlates of memory retrieval that suggest nontraditional processing roles for multiple distinct regions within posterior parietal cortex. *Journal of Neuroscience, 24,* 10084-10092.

Silberman, E. K., Putnam, F. W., Weingartner, H., Braun, B. G., & Post, R. M. (1985). Dissociative states in multiple personality disorder: A quantitative study. *Psychiatry Research, 15,* 253-260.

Spiegel, D., & Cardeña, E. (1991). Disintegrated experience: The dissociative disorders revisited. *Journal of Abnormal Psychology, 100,* 366-378.

Thapar, A., & McDermott, K. B. (2001). False recall and false recognition induced by presentation of associated words: Effects of retention interval and level of processing. *Memory & Cognition, 29,* 424-432.

Vanderlinden, J., Van Dyck, R., Vandereycken, W., & Vertommen, H. (1991). Dissociative experiences in the general population in Belgium and The Netherlands. An exploratory study with the Dissociation Questionnaire (Dis-Q). *Dissociation, 4,* 180-184.

Vanderlinden, J., Van Dyck, R., Vandereycken, W., Vertommen, H., & Verkes, R. J. (1993). The Dissociation Questionnaire (Dis-Q): Development and characteristics of a new self-report questionnaire. *Clinical Psychology and Psychotherapy, 1,* 21-28.

Veltman, D. J., de Ruiter, M. B., Rombouts, S. A. R. B., Lazeron, R. H. C., Barkhof, F., Van Dyck, R., Dolan, R. J., & Phaf, R. H. (2005). Neurophysiological correlates of increased verbal working memory in high-dissociative participants: A functional MRI study. *Psychological Medicine, 35,* 175-185.

doi:10.1300/J229v07n04_07

The Relationship Between Executive Attention and Dissociation in Children

Lisa DeMarni Cromer, PhD
Courtney Stevens, MS
Anne P. DePrince, PhD
Katherine Pears, PhD

SUMMARY. Dissociation involves disruption in the usually integrated functions of consciousness, memory, identity, and perception. Recent research with adults suggests that dissociation is associated with alterations in attention. Little work, however, has examined the attentional correlates of dissociation in childhood. This study is the first to investigate the specificity of cognitive functions related to dissociation in children. Twenty-four 5- to 8-year-old foster children completed several subtests of the NEPSY: A Developmental Neuropsychological Assessment (Korkman, Kirk, & Kemp, 1998) in the Executive Functioning/Attention domain. Foster caregivers completed the Child Dissociative Checklist (Bernstein & Putnam, 1986). Consistent with the adult

Lisa DeMarni Cromer and Courtney Stevens are affiliated with the University of Oregon.

Anne P. DePrince is affiliated with the University of Denver.

Katherine Pears is affiliated with the Oregon Social Learning Center.

Address corresponding to: Lisa DeMarni Cromer, Department of Psychology, 1227 University of Oregon, Eugene, OR 97403 (E-mail: ldemarni@uoregon.edu).

[Haworth co-indexing entry note]: "The Relationship Between Executive Attention and Dissociation in Children." Cromer, Lisa DeMarni et al. Co-published simultaneously in *Journal of Trauma & Dissociation* (The Haworth Medical Press, an imprint of The Haworth Press, Inc.) Vol. 7, No. 4, 2006, pp. 135-153; and: *Exploring Dissociation: Definitions, Development and Cognitive Correlates* (ed: Anne P. DePrince, and Lisa DeMarni Cromer) The Haworth Medical Press, an imprint of The Haworth Press, Inc., 2006, pp. 135-153. Single or multiple copies of this article are available for a fee from The Haworth Document Delivery Service [1-800-HAWORTH, 9:00 a.m. - 5:00 p.m. (EST). E-mail address: docdelivery@haworthpress.com].

literature, higher levels of childhood dissociation were associated with deficits in tasks requiring inhibition, but not with tasks requiring primarily planning, strategy, or multiple rule sets. doi:10.1300/J229v07n04_08 *[Article copies available for a fee from The Haworth Document Delivery Service: 1-800-HAWORTH. E-mail address: <docdelivery@haworthpress.com> Website: <http://www.HaworthPress.com> © 2006 by The Haworth Press, Inc. All rights reserved.]*

KEYWORDS. Dissociation, children, executive attention, inhibition

Dissociation involves a disruption in the usually integrated functions of consciousness, memory, identity, and perception (American Psychiatric Association, 2000). Dissociation often emerges during early childhood (Putnam, 1997) and is more common among individuals with a history of trauma or childhood abuse (Putnam, 1997; Silberg, 1998; Macfie, Cicchetti & Toth, 2001). Among abused children, dissociative behaviors can be adaptive as they might allow the child to maintain an appropriate and necessary attachment relationship with an abusive caregiver (Freyd, 1996). However, these same dissociative strategies, if not under conscious control, can be maladaptive for children in academic and other domains. One challenge for research on dissociation is to identify the cognitive correlates of dissociation early in development. Understanding specific cognitive processes that facilitate dissociation may guide differential diagnosis between dissociative and other disorders (e.g., Attention Deficit, Hyperactivity Disorder, ADHD), as well as provide leverage points for intervention efforts to facilitate successful functioning in non-threatening contexts.

While dissociation is well-described and identified in the literature, only a handful of studies have sought to empirically investigate the etiology (e.g., Macfie, Cicchetti & Toth, 2001) and cognitive mechanisms of dissociation (DePrince & Freyd, 1999, 2001, 2004; Dorahy, Middleton & Irwin, 2004; Dorahy, Irwin & Middleton, 2002; Elzinga, de Beurs, Sergeant, van Dyck, & Phaf, 2000). It is clearly established that there is a greater likelihood of finding dissociation in maltreated rather than in nonmaltreated children (e.g., Macfie et al., 2001; Putnam, 1997). Given the proposition that trajectories to pathological dissociation are established in childhood, close examination of specific cognitive correlates of dissociation in childhood should inform understanding of the developmental etiology of dissociation. Given that dissociation often develops in maltreated children, studying these cognitive correlates in foster children seems a good place to start. Cognitive inhibition is of particular interest in the literature review that follows. Cognitive inhibition encompasses a variety of tasks and constructs which have in common the ability to consciously exclude unwanted thoughts or stimuli.

In the last decade researchers have begun to examine cognitive correlates of dissociation using experimental and neuropsychological methods. This research has been conducted with college students (e.g., DePrince & Freyd, 1999) as well as individuals diagnosed with disorders associated with pathological levels of dissociation, including Dissociative Identity Disorder (DID; e.g., Dorahy et al., 2002) and Borderline Personality Disorder (BPD; e.g., Posner, Rothbart, Vizueta et al., 2002; see van der Hart, van der Kolk & Boon, 1998 and Wildgoose, Waller, Clarke, & Reid, 2000 for a discussion of the relationship between dissociation and BPD). Freyd et al. (1998) found that high dissociators in a college sample had increased interference during a color Stroop task (i.e., naming the color of ink used to print conflicting color words, as in the word 'green' written in blue ink). This suggests that high dissociators have greater difficulty inhibiting a task-irrelevant stimulus feature associated with a highly automatic response. Similarly, Dorahy et al. (2002) found weakened cognitive inhibition among patients diagnosed with DID in a negative priming experiment using words as stimuli; however, follow-up work has not found the same impairment when single digit numbers are used as stimuli (Dorahy et al., 2002, 2004). Posner and colleagues (Posner et al., 2002) also found evidence for weakened inhibition mechanisms in a group of sexually abused patients with Borderline Personality Disorder (BPD). These patients showed increased interference during a flanker task, in which participants indicated the direction a central arrow pointed while ignoring nearby, distracting arrows that could point in the same or opposite direction.

Taken together, these studies suggest that higher levels of dissociation are associated with deficits in the attentional mechanism of inhibition. Although the mechanism of inhibition has appeared under several different labels (e.g., conflict resolution, inhibitory control, interference-resolution, and executive control), tasks requiring either the suppression of a prepotent response or resistance to distracter interference have been considered part of the common construct of cognitive inhibition (Fan, Flombaum, McCandliss, Thomas, & Posner, 2003; Friedman & Miyake, 2004). Neuroimaging studies of diverse tasks requiring cognitive inhibition (e.g., Stroop, flanker, and go/no-go tasks) indicate a common set of overlapping brain regions involved across tasks, including the anterior cingulate and areas of prefrontal cortex, amidst large areas of task-specific activations (Fan et al. 2003; Jonides & Nee, 2004; Sylvester, Wager, Jonides, Lacey, Cheshin, & Nichols, 2003). Although the construct of inhibition itself is recognized as being non-unitary (e.g., Fan et al., 2003; Friedman & Miyake, 2004), it remains a useful way of describing a broad class of tasks.

In other attention domains, evidence suggests that high dissociators may be at a cognitive advantage relative to low dissociators. For example, DePrince and Freyd (1999) studied Stroop performance in a divided attention condition in which participants named the ink color while also studying the presented words in preparation for a memory test at the task's end. DePrince and Freyd reported a crossover interaction such that high dissociators showed greater Stroop interference under the typical selective attention condition, in which only the ink color was named, but reduced interference under divided attention conditions relative to low dissociators. This interaction suggested that high dissociators may be at a cognitive advantage under greater attentional load. Dorahy, Irwin, and Middleton (2004) summarized these findings with the suggestion that dissociation may mitigate the negative effects that increased demand on working memory would otherwise be expected to have on divided attention performance. Alternatively, de Ruiter and colleagues (this volume) offered the suggestion that high dissociators may benefit when cognitive task demands are high or more challenging.

In reviewing the child literature we were unable to identify any research examining dissociation in relation to performance on a neuropsychological assessment battery. However, Rogosch and Cicchetti (2005) used a children's version of the flanker task with a large group of children (N = 300) who had a range of maltreatment history and BDP characteristics to demonstrate that history of maltreatment did not influence flanker task performance. Interestingly, higher levels of BDP characteristics related to more interference (i.e., poorer inhibition of the flanking stimuli). Although dissociation was not directly measured in this study, the strong positive correlation between dissociation and BPD (e.g., van der Hart et al., 1996) suggests inhibitory mechanisms may also be deficient in highly dissociative children.

Attention condition has also been used to examine children's memory as a function of dissociation and trauma experience. Preschool children's memory for neutral and threat-related storybook pictures in either selective or dual attention conditions (Becker-Blease, Freyd &

Pears, 2004) was examined as a function of dissociation and maltreatment. In this study, abused/high dissociation children showed impaired recognition memory for threat-related pictures (relative to neutral pictures) in the divided attention condition relative to non-abused/low dissociation children. This supported the proposal that exposure to family violence and dissociation together may relate to changes in attention strategies, such as the use of divided attention, to keep threatening information out of awareness (Becker-Blease, Freyd & Pears, 2004).

Becker-Blease et al. (2004) made an important first step in examining the relationship of attention and dissociation in children. In extending this line of work, we made some methodological modifications. First, Becker-Blease and colleagues measured dissociation using a subscale of a trauma symptom checklist assessing absorption but not other symptoms of dissociation. Absorption likely reflected a less pathological facet of dissociation (see Brown et al., this volume for discussion). Second, their task combined attention and affective manipulations. This manipulation was helpful for studying the effects of attentional conditions on memory. However, just as the adult literature grapples with the conditions under which attentional correlates of dissociation are observed (e.g., Dorahy et al., 2004), the child literature would benefit from studies that consider the effects of dissociation on attention to and processing of emotion-neutral stimuli. Finally, a more thorough exploration of attentional and childhood dissociation will be aided by a more direct test of attention using reliable, standardized, and normed assessment tools that isolate different attention-related cognitive processes.

This study represents a preliminary and exploratory initiative to delineate the relationship between childhood dissociation and attention skills using a standardized assessment battery. Twenty-four 5- to 8-year-old foster children completed several subtests of the NEPSY: A Developmental Neuropsychological Assessment (Korkman, Kirk, & Kemp, 1998) in the Attention/Executive Functioning (AEF) domain. Scores on the NEPSY tasks were correlated with foster caregiver ratings of child dissociation based on the Child Dissociative Checklist (CDC; Bernstein & Putnam, 1986). Foster care children were selected for the study because they have been reported to have elevated average levels of dissociation (Putnam, 1997) and would be expected to represent a wider range of CDC scores than found in a community sample. Children in foster care also have high rates of neglect, abuse, and multiple traumas (Pears & Fisher, 2005).

Given the previous adult literature (DePrince & Freyd, 1999; Freyd et al., 1998), we predicted that higher levels of dissociation would be associated with poorer performance when tasks required inhibition. As indicated in Table 1, we assumed that the Knock and Tap and Auditory Attention Part A tasks required inhibition (see task descriptions below). This assumption was based on both the Nepsy manual, which indicates that Knock and Tap requires soley inhibition, and the attention literature, which defines inhibition as a necessary component of selective attention (Houghton, Tipper, Weaver, & Shore, 1996) required in the Auditory Attention Part A task. Task analyses for the remaining Nepsy attention spectrum tasks are also described in Table 1; testing the relationship between performance on these tasks and dissociation was exploratory.

METHOD

Participants

Twenty-four foster caregiver-child dyads in Lane County, Oregon were recruited through the local child welfare division. The children were part of a pilot for the Kids in Transition to School (KITS) Project, an intervention designed to increase the school readiness of children in foster care (Pears, Fisher & Bronz, 2006). This project was part of several ongoing foster care studies being conducted at the Oregon Social Learning Center (e.g, Fisher, Gunnar, Chamberlain, & Reid, 2000). Caseworkers were first approached and asked if foster caregivers could be contacted in order to offer participation in the study. If foster caregivers subsequently agreed to participate in the study, consent for the foster children to participate was obtained from the caseworkers (who represent the children's legal guardian the State of Oregon). Consent was received from all participating foster caregivers, and children provided assent. None of the recruited children declined to participate. Foster caregivers were paid $20 for their participation, and foster children received a small toy, juice and snack.

The sample of 24 children included 11 males ranging in age from 5.13 to 7.93 years ($M = 6.47$, $SD = .91$) and 13 females ranging in age from 4.99 to 8.48 years ($M = 6.62$, $SD = 1.12$). Twenty-one children were Caucasian, two were African American, and one was Native American. Because the study was a small pilot of an intervention focused primarily on promoting school readiness in children, practical constraints limited the ability to gather information on trauma history and clinical diagnoses information.

TABLE 1. Spearman's Rho Correlation Table of CDC Scores to NEPSY Scaled Scores with task analysis for subtests.

Subtest	Tower	Visual Search Faces	Auditory Attention	Auditory Response Set	Knock and Tap
Task Analysis per Nepsy Manual	Planning, Problem Solving, Monitoring	Speed & Accuracy	Inhibition+* & Selective Attention	Complex Cognitive Set & Set Shifting	Inhibition*
Child Dissociative Checklist	.07	.11	−.45*	−.16	−.58**
p	.73	.61	.03	.47	.003
Tower		−.11	−.03	−.26	−.10
p		.63	.88	.24	.65
Visual Attention Faces			−.25	−.35	−.49
p			.24	.10	.02
Auditory Attention				.80**	.36
p				.001	.09
Auditory Response Set					.49*
p					.02

significance* < .05 ** <.01
*Predicted deficit related to higher levels of dissociation.
+Indicates that although the NEPSY creators did not identify this subtest as a measure of inhibition, research indicates that by definition, inhibition is involved as a component of selective attention.

Measures

Child Dissociative Checklist. Dissociation was measured using the Child Dissociative Checklist (CDC), an observer-report measure used for screening children aged 5 to 18 (Bernstein & Putnam, 1986). The CDC measures children's dissociative behavior across a variety of contexts, including school, home, and play. An adult who is familiar with the child typically completes the CDC. The CDC has been shown to be reliable with a variety of different respondents including non-abusing parents, foster parents, and clinicians (Peterson & Putnam, 1994; Putnam, 1997). The CDC asks about a variety of child behaviors in the past 12 months, with responses being provided on a 3-point scale where 0 = "not true," 1 = "somewhat or sometimes true," and 2 = "very true." Summed scores in normal populations fall in the 2 to 3 point range out of a total possible 40 points. Scores in samples of maltreated children typically have a mean of 10.3 for 5- to 8-year-olds (Putnam, 1997). Children with Dissociative Disorder Not Otherwise Specified (DDNOS) and with Dissociative Identity Disorder (DID) typically have summed scale scores at least as high as 20 (Putnam, 1997). The internal consistency and test-retest reliability of the CDC is well established (Putnam et al., 1993; Wherry, Jolly & Feldman, 1994). Cronbach's alpha can be as high as .95 in large, diverse samples and in smaller samples, Cronbach's alpha is typically .73 with normal controls, .91 with sexually abused girls, and .80 with DID patients (Putnam et al., 1993). Split half reliabilities and test-retest reliabilities over one year are also high (Putnam et al., 1993). Good convergent validity has been established with a narrative dissociation assessment method (Macfie et al., 2001) and with therapist reports (Peterson & Putnam, 1994).

The NEPSY. Executive functions were assessed using the NEPSY, a standardized neuropsychological assessment instrument developed for use with children aged 3- to 12-years-old (Korkman, Kirk & Kemp, 1998). The NEPSY has been normed on a stratified sample of 1000 U.S. children of diverse ethnic backgrounds (50% female); good test-retest reliability, inter-rater reliability, and content validity have been demonstrated (Korkman, Kirk & Kemp, 1998). The NEPSY assesses five functional domains: Attention/Executive Functions, Language, Sensorimotor Functions, Visuospatial Processing, and Memory/Learning. The Attention/Executive Functions (AEF) core domain measures were used for the present study. The internal consistency and stability of the AEF subtests range from .83 to .87 for stratified age groups of 5 to 8 years. For the present study four subtests of the AEF domain were used, and the other NEPSY domains were not assessed. The four AEF tests administered, described in more detail below, included Tower, Visual Attention, Auditory Attention and Response Set, and Knock and Tap. Due to the age range of the sample, we did not administer two subtests (Statue and Design Fluency; Klenberg et al., 2001). The Tower subtest is a challenging task involving a variety of attention skills. It assesses planning, monitoring, self-regulation, and problem solving. This task involves a color picture as visual stimuli, three colored balls (yellow, red, blue) and three pegs fixed to a stationary board. For each trial, the child is to move the three colored balls, one at a time, using only one hand, so that the end result matches the stimulus picture. The child can use only a limited number of moves (as directed by the administrator) to recreate the stimulus picture. As inhibition is not implicated in Tower performance, no prediction was made regarding the association between dissociation and Tower performance.

The Visual Attention subtest is designed to assess attention in children as young as three. It measures the child's speed and accuracy for visually scanning an array of line drawings in order to locate and mark target drawings using a crayon. The subtest is scored by summing the number of correct targets, subtracting errors (incorrect targets), and factoring in speed (used for determining scaled score). In set A, the child locates a single style of cat amidst several other distracters (e.g., rabbit, flowers). In set B, the child must find two different faces from an assortment of similar other faces. There are 20 correct targets in each of set A and B, among 76 incorrect targets. Although set A and B of the visual attention task are typically collapsed into a single score (Korkman, Kirk & Kemp, 1998), these two variables were considered separately in the correlation analyses following previous work (Klenberg, Korkman & Nuuttila, 2001). Standard scores for the separate components were created using the same procedure as described below for the Auditory Attention measures. Neither the NEPSY manual (Korkman, Kirk & Kemp, 1998) nor the cognitive attention literature (Plude, Enns & Brodeur, 1994) consider visual search a task of inhibition. As inhibition is not implicated in visual search, no predictions were made regarding the correlation between dissociation and either set A or B of the visual attention task.

The Auditory Attention and Response Set tasks are typically collapsed into a single auditory attention and response set measure. More recent work has examined these scales separately (Klenberg, Korkman & Nuuttila, 2001) as they require different skill sets and represent varying levels of difficulty. Part A is relatively straightforward for children to perform. It is a three-minute continuous performance test of selective auditory attention (Korkman & Pesonen, 1994). It is considered to be "relatively simple and repetitive" (Korkman et al., 1998, p. 244). Part B is more challenging in that it requires the child to utilize a more complex cognitive set of skills including learning a new complex rule set, shifting sets, and regulating responses to contrasting stimuli (Klenberg et al., 2001; Korkman et al., 1998).

Both parts A and B require that the child listen and respond to an audiotape presentation of 180 words presented at 1 second intervals, for example "red . . . square . . . put . . . yellow . . . empty . . . thing . . . now." In part A the child is instructed to attend only to the word "red" and to place a red foam one inch square in a box lid upon each presentation. The child is provided with a haphazard pile of 16 blue, 14 yellow, 7 black, and 33 red squares from which to make a selection. The child is instructed, in part A, to ignore all other words and not to do anything at all until the word red is heard again. The child is allowed to practice twice while the test administrator reads a list of 11 words. If the child responds to the stimulus within one second, 2 points are scored, and within two or three seconds, 1 point is scored. There is a possible total score of 60 points (i.e., 30 targets) however commission errors, such as placing a blue tile in the box, result in the loss of 1 point. Scoring is done discretely so that the child does not get feedback. The tape plays continuously for 3 minutes without pause. Part A has a maximum score of 60. Because this is a measure of selective attention, of which inhibition is a necessary component (Houghton et al., 1996), we predicted a negative correlation to dissociation.

Part B immediately follows part A and the child is instructed to follow a new set of instructions. He or she must now put a yellow square in the box lid when s/he hears the word "red," do the opposite when hearing the word "yellow" by placing a red square in the box lid and follow a new rule when hearing the word "blue" by putting a blue square in the lid. Instructions further state that the child should do nothing upon hearing anything else at all. The child is permitted to practice twice to a list of 12 words that the administrator reads, before the auditory tape is played. Part B also consists of 180 words read at 1 second intervals. It contains 36 target words, 11 yellow, 11 red and 14 blue. Scoring is the same method as Part A. Part B has a maximum score of 72 points. We did not have a specific prediction for the relationship between dissociation and this task of complex cognitive sets.

In order to obtain separate scaled scores for both Parts A and B, we multiplied the raw score of Part A by 2.2 and Part B by 1.83 so that each of these subscales represented a score out of the maximum total 132 points. This approach is consistent with practices in the field to transform NEPSY scoring procedures to analyze separate parts of a subtest (see Perner, Kain & Barchfeld, 2002). From this value, a standard score was obtained from the NEPSY scoring manual. Analyses conducted on the untransformed raw scores had comparable results, but scaled scores were used to account for the expected performance differences due to age (Korkman et al., 1998; Klenberg et al., 2001).

Finally, the Knock and Tap subtest assesses the child's ability to inhibit behavioral impulses in response to visual stimuli that conflict with verbal directions (Korkman et al., 1998). In the first, most simple set, when the administrator knocks, the child must tap and vice versa. The child has several seconds to respond in each trial (where one knock or one tap equals a trial). In the second set, when the administrator makes a fist and taps with the side of her hand, the child must do a knock with her knuckles, and vice versa. When the administrator lays her hand flat on the table the child is told to do nothing at all and to keep the current hand position. As inhibition is implicated in this task, a negative relationship between dissociation and Knock and Tap performance was predicted.

Procedure

Foster caregivers completed the CDC in the Oregon Social Learning Center waiting room while child participants accompanied a test administrator to "play some games" and "win prizes." The NEPSY subtests were administered by trained clinical psychology doctoral students.

RESULTS

Dissociation

CDC scores in the sample ranged from 0 to 20, with a mean of 8.92 (SD = 5.74), Cronbach's alpha = .78. Compared to hundreds of normal controls (Putnam, 1997) the mean of this group is substantially higher (Cohen's d effect size = 1.9) but is comparable to samples of maltreated children (Putnam, 1997; Cohen's d effect size = 0.17). This suggests that although the sample of foster children is small, the range of dissociation scores expected among maltreated or neglected children are represented. CDC scores were distributed continuously across the 0 to 20 range, with no obvious grouping or divide between high and low dissociators. Past work examining the relationship of dissociation to attention has used larger samples and thus has been able to utilize only the high and low scores removing scores that were roughly within a standard deviation of the mean. Given the small sample size and the absence of an obvious break in scores, dissociation was treated as a continuous variable and correlation analyses were used.

Attention/Executive Functions

Scaled scores on the Tower task were normally distributed (M = 8.21, SD = 3.01). Most children scored at ceiling on the Cats visual attention subtest, so we did not include these in further analyses. Scaled scores on the second subtest of visual attention task (faces) had a moderate positive skew as did the Knock and Tap. Scaled scores on the auditory attention and response set subtest were normally distributed. We examined the two subtests separately as suggested in Klenberg et al. (2001). The scaled score for selective auditory attention was (M = 9.13, SD = 3.71) and for the more complex part B auditory response set (M = 7.5, SD = 2.38).

Correlations Between AEF and Dissociation

Table 1 presents correlations between the attention measures and CDC scores. Age was not controlled for in analyses as the scaled scores have factored age into the transformations from raw scores. Spearman's rho was used when calculating correlations for two reasons. First, there were up to two outliers on individual subscore measures and Person's r is sensitive to outliers. Second, the NEPSY uses scaled scores which transform the data into rank order data. Spearman's rho calculates correlations using rank ordered data and is therefore the appropriate test to use.

Of the three NEPSY subtests that were not classified as involving inhibition, there was no association between CDC scores and performance. The Tower, Visual Attention task, and Auditory Response Set all showed near-0 Spearman's rho correlations (see Table 1). It was predicted that dissociation would be negatively related to performance on the Knock and Tap, which requires inhibition. This hypothesis was supported, Spearman's rho = $-.58$, $p = .003$. This is considered a 'large' effect size. Inspection of the scatter plot revealed one far outlier. When this outlier was removed, the correlation remained significant, rho = $-.60$, $p = .003$. Because of the small sample size, we did not remove this outlier and report the more conservative score in the correlation table.

There was also a significant negative correlation between dissociation and Part A of the Auditory Attention Task, Spearman's rho = $-.45$, $p = .03$, which is a large effect size. As an internal validity check, we noted that performance on the two Auditory Attention Tasks was highly correlated, spearman's rho = $.77$, $p = .0001$. Because inhibition is thought to be a necessary component of selective attention (Houghton et al., 1996), we explored this selective attention relationship to dissociation using path analysis which allowed us to see if inhibition accounted for the effects of selective attention (Baron & Kenny, 1986). Using CDC score as the predicted variable in a regression model with Knock and Tap (inhibition) and auditory attention Part A (selective attention), we find that there is strong support for inhibition mediating the effect of the selective auditory attention. See Figure 1 for a model schematic.

FIGURE 1. Mediation Model of Inhibition, Selective Attention and Dissociation

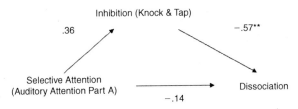

Inhibition (Knock & Tap)

.36   −.57**

Selective Attention
(Auditory Attention Part A)   ⟶   Dissociation
                                    −.14

The model shows that when Inhibtion/Knock and Tap is entered into a model mediating Selective Attention, the relationship between this task and dissociation is no longer significant.
**$p < .001$

DISCUSSION

This study examined the relationship between attention and dissociation in foster children. We had predicted a negative relationship between dissociation and performance on tasks requiring inhibition, as observed in the adult literature (DePrince & Freyd, 1999, 2001; Dorahy et al., 2002; Freyd et al., 1998). We also endeavored to expand this literature with exploratory analyses of other domains within attention, including visual search and planning. By using a standardized and normed neuropsychological assessment battery, we evaluated performance on five attention tasks tapping several facets of attention. We found no evidence for a relationship between dissociation and performance on tasks that required planning, problem solving and complex cognitive sets.

As predicted, higher levels of dissociation were associated with worse performance on Knock and Tap, a classic measure of inhibition. This finding is consistent with previous attention studies that demonstrated inhibition deficits in maltreated children with BPD characteristics (Rogosch & Cicchetti, 2005), adult DID patients (Dorahy et al., 2002), and high-dissociating college students (Freyd et al., 1998). That we replicated findings of inhibition deficits with a sample of young children doing developmentally appropriate tasks suggests that the inhibition/dissociation relationship may have its origins early in development.

A strong negative relationship was also observed between dissociation and Auditory Attention performance. The NEPSY manual identifies this task as a selective Auditory Attention Task. However, during test administration, we noted that this auditory attention measure behaviorally could be likened to a go/no-go task, which is a common measure of inhibition. In a go/no-go task, the same response (placing a red square in the container) is given for the 'go' stimulus (the word 'red') and inhibited for all other stimuli (the words 'yellow,' 'blue,' 'put,' etc.). The child must respond only to the word 'red,' and inhibit responses to all other stimuli. As indicated in the attention literature, inhibition is a necessary component of selective attention. Therefore this strong relationship between the Auditory Attention and dissociation was not surprising. In utilizing the Baron and Kenny (1986) path analysis technique, we were able to essentially partial out the effect of inhibition and found that selective attention no longer significantly predicted dissociation. This modeling lends further support for the relationship between inhibition and dissociation. We acknowledge however, that inhibition is an ill-defined word in the cognitive literature (see MacLeod, Dodd, Sheard, Wilson, & Bibi, 2003 for review). In the present analyses we are taking the position of MacLeod et al. (2003) that "inhibition" which some have posited is synonymous with selective attention (e.g., Houghton et al., 1996) actually has several meanings and likely is a component of, yet not the same as, selective attention.

Despite the negative relationship between dissociation and auditory attention, we did not find a similar relationship with the Auditory Response Set task, a test requiring complex rule sets and set shifting. Success at this task may be explained by the use of organizational strategies (see MacLeod et al., 2003) rather than inhibitory abilities. Dissociation was also not related to children's performance on visual search and tower tasks. This suggests that dissociation is not associated with a pervasive impairment in cognitive performance in the general attention/executive functioning domain as measured by the NEPSY. Further study will be needed, however, in order to more broadly assess cognitive differences related to dissociation.

These findings support DePrince and Freyd's (1999) speculation that individuals may develop alternative cognitive styles in order to accommodate dissociative tendencies. Our data point to strong relationships between dissociation and inhibition in the absence of other deficits (e.g., planning) in children as young as 5-8 years. Over time, dissociative children may compensate for inhibition deficits as other cognitive functions develop (e.g., complex cognitive sets, set shifting), creating a set of skills that appear to be relative strengths. Though we cannot test this longitudinal hypothesis in the current data set, this proposition is supported by the literature on neuroplasticity. Such research documents that, in the face of deficits in some areas, compensatory strengths can develop in other domains (e.g., Bavelier, Tomann, Hutton, Mitchell, Corina, Liu, et al., 2000; Neville & Bavelier, 2002; Stevens & Neville, 2006). Therefore, skill development in other aspects of attention may help dissociative children compensate for relative difficulties in inhibition over time.

This fits with DePrince and Freyd's (1999) observation that high dissociators show decreased interference under divided attention conditions relative to selective, compared to low dissociators. Further, recent intervention studies have demonstrated the malleability of attention following specific training activities (Green & Bavalier, 2003; Rueda, Rothbart, McCandliss, Saccomanno, & Posner, 2005). Thus, the possibility that early effects of dissociation may lead to adaptations in cognitive style over time is an exciting area for future study.

Clinical Relevance

From a clinical intervention perspective, treatment models for dissociative pathology center on an executive function (EF) framework (e.g., Hornstein, 1998; Putnam, 1997; Silberg, 1998). In treating severely pathologically dissociative children (with DID), clinicians train the child and the child's family to give the child executive control over his or her alter personalities. For example, the clinicians may refuse to talk to any of the alter personalities and require the child to act as a go-between for the alter personalities and the clinician. Thus, this therapy teaches the child to master several EFs. Specifically, the child must learn to control cognitive shifting between alters so that he or she can be present with the clinician; the child learns to inhibit the voices of alter personalities; and the child learns emotional self-control and organizational skills as the executive cognitive functions are trained and developed. Therefore, from a clinical level of observation, we see an apparent relationship between EF and dissociation, through which EF is increased while dissociation decreases.

Differential Diagnosis

A clear understanding of the cognitive correlates of child dissociation may aid in improving differential diagnosis of dissociative disorders in clinical populations. Dissociative disorders often go undiagnosed or co-present with other conditions such as anxiety, mood, and conduct disorders (Hornstein, 1998; Peterson, 1998; Ross, 1996; Silberg, 1998) as well as ADHD (Peterson, 1998; Silberg, 1998). In comparing the present study to studies evaluating attention performance of children diagnosed with ADHD we find critical differences. In a meta-analytic review of 83 ADHD studies, Willcutt and colleagues (Willcutt, Doyle, Nigg, Faraone, & Pennington, 2005) found that ADHD children did poorly on inhibition (comparable to NEPSY Knock and Tap), set shifting (comparable to NEPSY auditory part B), and planning (Tower tasks). These data point to common deficits in inhibition between high dissociation and ADHD samples however the patterns diverge for planning/complex tasks. The current findings point to the possibility that dissociation and ADHD could be differentiated by performance on planning/complex tasks. Thus, this study points to the value of additional, larger scale studies designed to identify difference in cognitive performance between highly dissociative children and children diagnosed with ADHD.

Limitations of the Present Study

There were several limitations to the present study. First, the small sample size limits both power for and choice of statistical analyses. Previous research relied on group comparisons of high versus low dissociators; however, we were unable to do such comparisons, as we had a consistent range of CDC cores from 0 to 20 without an obvious cut point. Between group comparisons would have required that we remove participants whose CDC scores were about one standard deviation on either side of the mean, and this would have reduced our sample size and thus our statistical power. Second, child maltreatment data were not collected for this sample. We assumed that many if not all of the children entered foster care because of some form of maltreatment or neglect. However, we were unable to examine the relationship between chronicity or severity of maltreatment and neuropsychological performance.

Future Directions

This study provides exciting directions for future research. First, this study provides clear justification for future empirical work examining the association between neuropsychological function and dissociation with larger samples of foster children. Second, future studies should collect information about maltreatment exposure, clinical diagnoses, length of time in foster care, and other responses to trauma (beyond dissociation). Ultimately, as we look to the future, we hope that specific attention "leverage points" can be identified as particular deficits and strengths for highly dissociative children. By delineating cognitive environments that either enhance or improve performance as a function of dissociation, educational interventions can be designed to support dissociative children's academic success.

REFERENCES

American Psychiatric Association. (2000). *Diagnostic and statistical manual of mental disorders (4th ed., text revision)*. Washington, DC: Author.

Baron, R., & Kenny, D. A. (1986). The moderator-mediator variable distinction in social psychological research: Conceptual, strategic, and statistical considerations. *Journal of Personality and Social Psychology, 51(6)*, 1173-1182.

Bavelier, D., Brozinsky, C., Tomann, A., Mitchell, T., Corina, D., Liu, G., et al. (2001). Impact of early deafness and early exposure to sign language on the cerebral organization for motion processing. *Journal of Neuroscience, 21(22)*, 8931-8942.

Becker-Blease, K.A., Freyd, J.J., Pears, K.C. (2004). Preschoolers' memory for threatening information depends on trauma history and attentional context: Implications for the development of dissociation. *Journal of Trauma and Dissociation, 5*, 113-131.

Bernstein, E., & Putnam, F.W. (1986). Development, reliability and validity of a dissociation scale. *Journal of Nervous and Mental Disease, 174*, 727-735.

Brown, R.J. (2006). Different types of dissociation have different psychological mechanisms. *Journal of Trauma and Dissociation, 7(4)*, 7-28.

DePrince, A.P., & Freyd, J.J. (1999). Dissociative tendencies, attention, and memory. *Psychological Science, 10(5)*, 449-452.

DePrince, A.P., & Freyd, J.J. (2001). Memory and dissociative tendencies: The roles of attentional context and word meaning in a direct forgetting task. *Journal of Trauma and Dissociation, 2(2)*, 67-82.

DePrince, A.P., & Freyd, J.J. (2004). Forgetting trauma stimuli. *Psychological Science, 15(7)*, 488-492.

de Ruiter, M.B., Elzinga, B.M., & Phaf, R.H. (2006). Dissociation: Cognitive capacity or dysfunction? *Journal of Trauma and Dissociation, 7(4)*, 115-134.

Dorahy, M.J., Irwin, H.J., & Middleton, W. (2002). Cognitive inhibition in Dissociative Identity Disorder (DID): Developing an understanding of working memory function in DID. *Journal of Trauma and Dissociation, 3(3)*, 111-132.

Dorahy, M.J., Irwin, H.J., & Middleton, W. (2004). Assessing markers of working memory function in Dissociative Identity Disorder using neutral stimuli: A comparison with clinical and general population samples. *Australian and New Zealand Journal of Psychiatry, 38*, 47-55.

Elzinga, B.M., de Beurs, E., Sergeant, J.A., Van Dyck, R., & Phaf, R.H. (2000). Dissociative style and directed forgetting. *Cognitive Therapy and Research, 24(3)*, 279-295.

Fan, J., Flombaum, J.I., McCandliss, B.D., Thomas, K.M., & Posner, M.I. (2003). Cognitive and brain consequences of conflict. *NeuroImage, 18(1)*, 42-5.

Freyd, J.J. (1996). *Betrayal trauma: The logic of forgetting childhood abuse.* Cambridge, Massachusetts: Harvard University Press.

Freyd, J.J., Martorello, S.R., Alvarado, J.S., Hayes, A.E., & Christman, J.C. (1998). Cognitive environments and dissociative tendencies: Performance on the standard Stroop task for high versus low dissociators. *Applied Cognitive Psychology, 12,* S91-S103.

Friedman, N.P., & Miyake, A. (2004). The relations among inhibition and interference control functions: A latent variable analysis. *Journal of Experimental Psychology: General, 133,* 101-135.

Green, C., & Bavelier, D. (2003). Action video game modifies visual attention. *Nature, 423,* 534-537.

Hornstein, N.L. (1998). Complexities of psychiatric differential diagnosis of children with dissociative symptoms and disorders. In J.L. Silberg (Ed.), *The dissociative child: Diagnosis, treatment, and management* (2nd ed.), pp. 27-45. Lutherville, Maryland: Sidran Press.

Houghton, G., Tipper, S.P., Weaver, B., & Shore, D.I. (1996). Inhibition and interference in selective attention: Some tests of a neural network model. *Visual Cognition, 3(2),* 119-14.

Jonides, J., & Nee, D.E. (2004). Resolving conflict in mind and brain. *American Psychological Association Science Briefs, 18,* accessed 3/17/06 http://www.apa.org/science/psa/sb-jonides.html.

Klenberg, L., Korkman, M., & Lahti-Nuuttila, P. (2001). Differential development of attention and executive functions in 3- to 12-year-old Finnish children. *Developmental neuropsychology, 20(1),* 407-428.

Korkman, M., Kirk, U., & Kemp, S. (1998). *NEPSY: A developmental neuropsychological assessment manual.* San Antonio, Texas: Harcourt Bruce & Company.

Korkman, M., & Pesonen, A. (1994). A comparison of neuropsychological test profiles of children with Attention Deficit-Hyperactivity Disorder and/or Learning Disorder. *Journal of Learning Disabilities, 27(6),* 383-392.

Liotti, G. (2006). A model of dissociation based on attachment theory and research. *Journal of Trauma and Dissociation, 7(4),* 55-73.

Macfie, J., Cicchetti, D., & Toth, S.L. (2001). The development of dissociation in maltreated preschool-aged children. *Development and Psychopathology, 13,* 233-254.

MacLeod, C.M., Dodd, M.D., Sheard, E.D., Wilson, D.E., & Bibi, U. (2003). In opposition to inhibition. *The Psychology of Learning and Motivation, 43,* 163-214.

Neville, H.J., & Bavelier, D. (2002). Cross-modal plasticity: Where and how? *Nature Reviews Neuroscience, 3,* 443-452.

Pears, K., & Fisher, P. (2005). Developmental, cognitive, and neuropsychological functioning in preschool-aged Foster Children: Associations with prior maltreatment placement history. *Developmental and Behavioral Pediatrics, 26(2),* 112-122.

Perner, J., Kain, W., & Barchfeld, P. (2002). Executive control and higher-order theory of mind in children as risk of ADHD. *Infant and Child Development, 11,* 141-158.

Peterson, G. (1998). Diagnostic taxonomy: Past to future. In J.L. Silberg (Ed.), *The dissociative child: Diagnosis, treatment, and management* (2nd ed.), pp. 3-26. Lutherville, Maryland: Sidran Press.

Peterson, G., & Putnam, F.W. (1994). Preliminary results of the field trial of proposed criteria for dissociative disorder of childhood. *Dissociation, 8(4)*, 212-220.

Plude, D., Enns, J., & Brodeur, D. (1994). The development of selective attention: A life-span overview. *Acta Psychologica, 86*, 227-272.

Posner, M.I., Rothbart, M.K., Vizueta, N., Levy, K.N., Evans, D., Thomas, K., & Clarkin, J.F. (2002). Attentional mechanisms of borderline personality disorder. *Proceedings of the National Academy of the Sciences of the United States of America, 99(25).*

Putnam, F.W., Helmers, K., & Trickett, P.K. (1993). Development, reliability, and validity of a child dissociative scale. *Child Abuse and Neglect, 17*, 731-741.

Putnam, F.W. (1997). *Dissociation in children and adolescents: A developmental perspective.* New York: The Guildford Press.

Rogosch, F.A., & Cicchetti, D. (2005). Child maltreatment, attention networks, and potential precursors to borderline personality disorder. *Development and Psychopathology, 17*, 1071-1089.

Ross, C. (1996). History, phenomenology, and epidemiology of dissociation. In L.K. Michelson & W.J. Ray (Eds.), *Handbook of dissociation: Theoretical, empirical, and clinical perspectives* (pp. 3-24). New York, NY: Plenum Press.

Rueda, M.R., Rothbart, M., McCandliss, B., Saccomanno, L., & Posner, M.I. (2005). Training, maturation, and genetic influences on the development of executive attention. *Proceedings of the National Academy of Sciences of the U.S.A., 102*, 14931-14936.

Silberg, J.L. (Ed.) (1998). *The dissociative child: Diagnosis, treatment, and management* (2nd ed.). Lutherville, Maryland: Sidran Press.

Stevens, C., & Neville, H. (2006). Neuroplasticity as a double-edged sword: Deaf enhancements and dyslexic deficits in motion processing. *Journal of Cognitive Neuroscience, 18*, 701-714.

Sylvester, C.C., Wager, T.D., Jonides, J., Lacey, S.C., Cheshin., A., and Nichols, T.E. (2003). Processes of interference resolution as revealed by functional magnetic resonance imaging. 2003 *Meeting of Cognitive Neuroscience Society.*

van der Hart, O., van der Kolk, B.A., & Boon, S. (1998). The treatment of dissociative disorders. In D.J. Bremner & C.R. Marmar (Eds.).*Trauma, memory, and dissociation.* Washington, DC, US: American Psychiatric Association, 253-283.

Wherry, J.N., Jolly, J.B., Feldman, J., Adam, B., & Manjanatha, S. (1994). The Child Dissociative Checklist: Preliminary findings of a screening instrument. *Journal of Child Sexual Abuse, 3*, 51-66.

Wildgoose, A., Waller, G., Clarke, S., & Reid, A. (2000). Psychiatric symptomatology in borderline and other personality disorders: Dissociation and fragmentation as mediators. *Journal of Nervous and Mental Diseases, 188(11)*, 757-763.

Willcutt, E.G., Doyle, A.E., Nigg, J.T., Faraone, S.V., & Pennington, B.F. (2005). Validity of the Executive Function Theory of Attention-Deficit/Hyperactivity Disorder: A meta-analytic review. *Biological Psychiatry, 57*, 1336-1346.

doi:10.1300/J229v07n04_08

Index

BOOK ORDER FORM!

Order a copy of this book with this form or online at:
http://www.HaworthPress.com/store/product.asp?sku= 5988

Exploring Dissociation
Definitions, Development and Cognitive Correlates

—— in softbound at $28.00 ISBN-13: 978-0-7890-3327-7 / ISBN-10: 0-7890-3327-5.
—— in hardbound at $59.00 ISBN-13: 978-0-7890-3326-0 / ISBN-10: 0-7890-3326-7.

COST OF BOOKS _____

POSTAGE & HANDLING _____
US: $4.00 for first book & $1.50
for each additional book
Outside US: $5.00 for first book
& $2.00 for each additional book.

SUBTOTAL _____

In Canada: add 6% GST. _____

STATE TAX _____
CA, IL, IN, MN, NJ, NY, OH, PA & SD residents
please add appropriate local sales tax.

FINAL TOTAL _____
If paying in Canadian funds, convert
using the current exchange rate,
UNESCO coupons welcome.

❏ **BILL ME LATER:**
Bill-me option is good on US/Canada/
Mexico orders only; not good to jobbers,
wholesalers, or subscription agencies.

❏ **Signature** _____

❏ **Payment Enclosed: $**_____

❏ **PLEASE CHARGE TO MY CREDIT CARD:**

❏ Visa ❏ MasterCard ❏ AmEx ❏ Discover
❏ Diner's Club ❏ Eurocard ❏ JCB

Account #_____

Exp Date_____

Signature_____
(Prices in US dollars and subject to change without notice.)

PLEASE PRINT ALL INFORMATION OR ATTACH YOUR BUSINESS CARD

Name

Address

City   State/Province   Zip/Postal Code

Country

Tel   Fax

E-Mail

May we use your e-mail address for confirmations and other types of information? ❏Yes ❏No We appreciate receiving
your e-mail address. Haworth would like to e-mail special discount offers to you, as a preferred customer.
We will never share, rent, or exchange your e-mail address. We regard such actions as an invasion of your privacy.

Order from your **local bookstore** or directly from
The Haworth Press, Inc. 10 Alice Street, Binghamton, New York 13904-1580 • USA
Call our toll-free number (1-800-429-6784) / Outside US/Canada: (607) 722-5857
Fax: 1-800-895-0582 / Outside US/Canada: (607) 771-0012
E-mail your order to us: orders@HaworthPress.com

For orders outside US and Canada, you may wish to order through your local
sales representative, distributor, or bookseller.
For information, see http://HaworthPress.com/distributors

(Discounts are available for individual orders in US and Canada only, not booksellers/distributors.)

Please photocopy this form for your personal use.
www.HaworthPress.com

 BOF06